Why Poison Ourselves?
A Precautionary Approach
to Synthetic Chemicals

ANNE PLATT McGINN

Chris Bright, *Editor*

WORLDWATCH PAPER 153

November 2000

THE WORLDWATCH INSTITUTE is an independent, nonprofit environmental research organization in Washington, DC. Its mission is to foster a sustainable society in which human needs are met in ways that do not threaten the health of the natural environment or future generations. To this end, the Institute conducts interdisciplinary research on emerging global issues, the results of which are published and disseminated to decision-makers and the media.

FINANCIAL SUPPORT for the Institute is provided by the Compton Foundation, the Geraldine R. Dodge Foundation, the Ford Foundation, the Richard & Rhoda Goldman Fund, the William and Flora Hewlett Foundation, W. Alton Jones Foundation, Charles Stewart Mott Foundation, the Curtis and Edith Munson Foundation, David and Lucile Packard Foundation, John D. and Catherine T. MacArthur Foundation, Summit Foundation, Turner Foundation, U.N. Population Fund, Wallace Genetic Foundation, Wallace Global Fund, Weeden Foundation, and the Winslow Foundation. The Institute also receives financial support from its Council of Sponsors members—Tom and Cathy Crain, Roger and Vicki Sant, Robert Wallace and Raisa Scriabine, and Eckart Wintzen—and from the many Friends of Worldwatch.

THE WORLDWATCH PAPERS provide in-depth, quantitative and qualitative analysis of the major issues affecting prospects for a sustainable society. The Papers are written by members of the Worldwatch Institute research staff and reviewed by experts in the field. Regularly published in five languages, they have been used as concise and authoritative references by governments, nongovernmental organizations, and educational institutions worldwide. For a partial list of available Papers, see back pages.

The views expressed are those of the author and do not necessarily represent those of the Worldwatch Institute; of its directors, officers, or staff; or of its funding organizations.

Table of Contents

Introduction 5

Toxics and the Precautionary Principle 10

Pulp and Paper: Designing the Toxic Out of the System . . 18

Pesticides: Substituting Knowledge for Synthetics 29

PVC: Turning Complex Problems into Multiple
    Opportunities. 47

Leveraging Change 61

Notes 73

Tables and Figures

Table 1: *The UNEP "Dirty Dozen" POPs* 9

Table 2: *Average Range of Chemical Pulp Mill Effluent by Region* . . . 24

Table 3: *Integrated Pest Management and Integrated
    Vector Management: Selected Parallels* 44

Table 4: *Alternatives to Major Construction Uses of PVC, According
    to a 1997 Canadian Study* 58

Table 5: *Selected International Conventions Complementary
    to the POPs Treaty* 64

Table 6: *Regulatory Status of the "Dirty Dozen" POPs* 66

Figure 1: *Where POPs Fit in the Commercial Chemical Universe* 15

Figure 2: *World Paper Production, by Fiber Supply, 1961–97* 20

Figure 3: *World Production of ECF, TCF, and Elemental
    Chlorine (EC) Pulp, 1990–99* 26

Figure 4: *Pesticide Exports and Imports in Industrial and Developing Countries, 1961–98* 35

Figure 5: *Global Count of Pesticide Resistant Species, 1908–98* 37

Figure 6: *PVC Consumption by Region, 1991–2001 (estimated); and PVC Production Capacity, Regional Percentages, 1999* 48

Figure 7: *Changes in Toxic Chemical Use Per Product Unit, Reported Under the Massachusetts Toxics Use Reduction Act, 1990–97* 69

ACKNOWLEDGMENTS: Many thanks to the following individuals for their review comments: Bill Carroll, Rutherford Platt (my Dad), Romeo Quijano, Ted Schettler, Joe Thornton, and Joel Tickner. Thanks also to Joseph LaDou, Warren Muir, Elizabeth Nesbitt, and Jack Weinberg for their thoughts on the general argument, and to Charlotte Brody, Pat Costner, Clif Curtis, Lynn Goldman, Liz Harriman, Tony Jaegel, Rich Liroff, David Pimentel, and Larry Yates for clarifying key points and data.

Many people at Worldwatch contributed to this project. I would especially like to thank my editor and colleague, Chris Bright, who kept this unconventional project on track and on time. Special thanks also to Hilary French for her insightful comments and support; to Brian Halweil, Ashley Mattoon, and Payal Sampat, who contributed key data and salient comments on the drafts, to Lori Baldwin Brown, Jonathan Guzman, and Joseph Gravely who together made sure my sources were up-to-date and in hand; and to Janet Abramovitz and Lisa Mastny for their reviews. I am grateful to interns Ann Hwang, who tracked down volumes of information and gave me a crash course on organic chemistry, and to Sarah Porter, who contributed research in 1999. Thanks also to those who produced and oversaw the outreach of this project, especially Liz Doherty, who kept a tight ship on time with her usual style and finesse; and Dick Bell, Denise Warden, and Niki Clark. Lastly, heartfelt thanks to my husband and son for everything.

ANNE PLATT McGINN is a Senior Researcher at Worldwatch Institute, where she researches marine and environmental health issues. She is a regular contributor to the Institute's annual publications, *State of the World* and *Vital Signs*, and bi-monthly magazine, *World Watch*. Her last contribution to this series was Worldwatch Paper 145, *Safeguarding the Health of Oceans*.

Introduction

Nothing could be more ordinary than plastic. Plastic bags and plastic pens, the plastic in our computers and cars: this material has become a basic element of our built environment. And the same could be said for many other types of synthetic chemicals. Synthetics surround us in all sorts of ways. Even if you wanted to, it would be impossible to withdraw from their embrace. You might not be caught dead in a polyester shirt, for example, but the 100 percent cotton fabric that you might prefer is likely to have come from a field treated with synthetic pesticides. Your furniture may be wood and fabric, but it was probably manufactured with synthetic solvents, glues, and coatings. Cinema and recorded music are products of synthetic materials. The computer revolution is based on the synthetic chemical revolution that preceded it. And you very likely know a few people who owe their lives to medical procedures that depend on all kinds of synthetics, from the materials used in surgical equipment to the drugs prescribed. Perhaps that's true of you personally.

Synthetics are now so pervasive—so ordinary—that it can be difficult to see how profoundly they have changed human life. Yet mass production of these materials is a relatively recent development. The technology has its origins in mid-19th century European laboratories, where chemists were beginning to create completely novel organic compounds—for example, various anesthetics and disinfectants. (An organic compound is a chemical that contains carbon.) DDT, arguably the world's most famous pesticide, dates from this era; it was synthesized in 1874 by a German chemistry student, although its pesticidal properties were not appreciated until the 1930s. The first plastics were synthesized from cellulose (the primary constituent of wood) in the 1890s. The key to our current form of mass production was discovered at about the same time, when chemists realized that they didn't have to use plant products such as cellulose as their raw material. Synthetics could be produced directly from oil. By 1900, oil-based synthetics had revolutionized a major industry—the production of dyes—and the Age of Synthetics had dawned.[1]

During the first half of the 20th century, synthetics flooded one manufacturing process after another, since they were often much cheaper than such traditional materials as rubber, wood, metal, glass, and plant fiber. In some cases the synthetic displaced a traditional material outright. Vinyl, for instance, was developed in the 1920s as a rubber substitute. During World War II, it helped ease the demand for this essential plant product; tires still had to be made of rubber, but vinyl worked well as a wire insulator. Just as important, however, has been the interest in combining old and new— the metal that has a specialty coating to make it more durable, the flooring laminate composed of resin and wood fiber, and so forth. Today, synthetic organic chemicals flow through just about every pipe in the chemical economy.[2]

Yet despite its extraordinary success, the synthetic chemical economy is a profoundly mysterious enterprise— even for professional chemists. Scientists have learned how to transform oil into a vast array of extremely useful materials. But they have also learned that the production, use, and disposal of these materials can inflict very serious damage— damage that has generally been unexpected and that has occasionally been horrible. In Bhopal, India, some 16,000 people died and hundreds of thousands were injured after the 1984 methyl isocyanate gas leak at a Union Carbide pesticide plant. Recent studies from various places—including the Netherlands, the United States, and Arctic Quebec—have discovered health problems in children exposed to very low levels of toxic synthetics in the womb or through nursing. Such children were found to suffer from more frequent ear and respiratory infections, and from delayed development, both physical and mental. Chronic exposure to such materials is injuring wildlife as well. In the North American Great Lakes, for example, various species of birds and fish still exhibit poor reproduction and physical deformities caused by exposure to a variety of dangerous synthetics that have haunted the region's soil and water for decades. These and many other places are suffering from the "external," largely uncounted costs of synthetic chemical use.[3]

There are today probably between 50,000 and 100,000 synthetic chemicals in commercial production, and new synthetics are entering commerce at an average rate of three per day. These numbers appear to suggest a high degree of "collective confidence" in our ability to handle synthetic materials. And yet, from an environmental perspective, one simple question hangs over the whole enterprise: what will these chemicals eventually do—to people, and to the environment in general? Despite all the literature that has accumulated on this subject over the past four or five decades, the answer to this question is depressingly simple: we really don't know. We are struggling to invent methods for assessing the risks from our *current* levels of synthetics exposure— even as more and more synthetics pour into the market. No doubt, many synthetics are benign. But roughly a century after the synthetic revolution began, it's still common to synthesize first and ask the hard questions later—and that's asking for trouble.[4]

There is now an important opportunity to rethink our approach to synthetic chemicals. In early 2001, a treaty on a class of dangerous synthetics known as "persistent organic pollutants," or POPs, is scheduled to be concluded. (POPs are defined in detail in the next section.) The treaty is known officially as "The International Legally Binding Instrument for Implementing International Action on Certain Persistent Organic Pollutants," and it was organized under the auspices of the U.N. Environment Programme (UNEP). Its text was developed over the course of more than two years by officials from over 120 nations, with the advice of hundreds of non-governmental organizations (NGOs) and independent scientists. The result is a document that singles out 12 chemicals or chemical groups for high priority action. Several of them have been banned in industrial countries for years. The POPs that made this "dirty dozen" list include nine pesticides, one group of compounds used primarily as liquid insulators in transformers (polychlorinated biphenyls, or PCBs), and two closely related chemical groups that are the byproducts of many industrial processes (dioxins and furans). (See Table 1.)[5]

In June 1998, when negotiations on the treaty began, UNEP Executive Director Klaus Töpfer declared that "the ultimate goal must be the elimination of POPs, not simply their better management." An optimistic assessment of the negotiations might see the treaty moving towards that goal. In September 1999, the treaty parties agreed to list eight of the dirty dozen chemicals on Annex A, which calls for their eventual elimination. Many participants also argue that the treaty should apply to other POPs, besides those on the dirty dozen list. Yet there is no firm agreement on how many chemicals should be considered in this group. A conservative reckoning would fix that number at several dozen, but other estimates run into the hundreds or thousands. And there may be hundreds of other chemicals that are similar to POPs, but that don't fully fit within the strict definition; these too would presumably be candidates for a phase-out. Given our uncertainty over the risks entailed by many synthetics, and given the rate at which new synthetics are introduced, it's difficult to see the treaty's chemical-by-chemical approach as a comprehensive solution. Clearly, other kinds of efforts will be needed as well.[6]

This paper adopts a perspective very different from that of the treaty, not as a replacement of the treaty, but as an essential supplement to it. The treaty is aimed at only a handful of the most spectacularly troublesome chemicals (although it's true that it may eventually be expanded to include other chemicals). But the precedents for even this rather modest approach aren't very favorable. Several

TABLE 1

The UNEP "Dirty Dozen" POPs

Persistent Organic Pollutant	Date of Introduction	Definition and Primary Applications
Aldrin	1949	Insecticide used against soil pests (primarily termites) on corn, cotton, and potatoes.
Chlordane	1945	Insecticide now used primarily for termite control.
DDT	1942	Insecticide now used mainly against mosquitoes.
Dieldrin	1948	Insecticide used on fruit, soil, and seed crops, including corn, cotton, and potatoes.
Endrin	1951	Rodenticide and insecticide used on cotton, rice, and corn.
Heptachlor	1948	Insecticide used against soil insects, especially termites. Also used against fire ants and mosquitoes.
Hexachloro-benzene	1945	Fungicide. Also a byproduct of pesticide manufacturing and a contaminant of other pesticide products.
Mirex	1959	Insecticide used on ants and termites. One of the most stable and persistent pesticides. Also a fire retardant.
Toxaphene	1948	Insecticide used especially against ticks and mites. A mixture of up to 670 chemicals.
PCBs	1929	Used primarily in capacitors and trans-formers, and in hydraulic and heat transfer systems. Also used in weatherproofing, carbonless copy paper, paint, adhesives, and plasticizers in synthetic resins.
Dioxins	1920s	Byproducts of combustion (especially of plastics) and of chlorine product manufacturing and paper bleaching.
Furans	1920s	Byproducts, especially of PCB manufacturing, often with dioxins.

Source: See endnote 5.

European countries have mandated reductions in POPs or POP-like compounds, and have made little progress. For example, the eight nations party to the 1990 North Sea Conference agreed to destroy all PCBs by 1999 but have not done so. (The conference was one of a series of forums on North Sea management, but not a treaty.)[7]

The POPs treaty's assumption appears to be that the standard, chemical-by-chemical approach is still workable, despite its failure to ask basic questions about the industry's tendency to produce dangerous materials. The assumption in this paper is that the standard approach amounts to a necessary but not a sufficient condition for significant change. Quantum improvement is not likely until some basic questions *are* asked—by policy makers, by business people, and by the public in general.

Is it possible to "detoxify" the economy without crippling its productive capacity? This is the line of inquiry pursued here, by examining three very different industries: the manufacture of paper, pesticides, and the plastic known as polyvinylchloride, or PVC. These industries have been chosen not because they offer an exhaustive picture of the entire chemical economy, but because they are representative of the problems and opportunities within it. Each is a major sector through which toxic chemicals move. Each covers a broad economic "cross-section," which may include manufacturing, retail, disposal issues, and relationships with allied industries. Each is responding to a general global demand for its products. And each offers an important point of leverage for changing the chemical economy as a whole.

Toxics and the Precautionary Principle

The chemical industry's problem with toxics is perhaps best approached by looking first at the toxics themselves. It's useful to begin with a definition of "POP." Take the terms that make up the name one at a time:

"P" as in persistent: POPs are very stable.

POPs do not break down readily under normal natural conditions. Because of their stability, POPs will remain in the environment for decades after they are released. Over this span of time, they are likely to travel great distances, especially since many of them are prone to mobility. Many POPs evaporate at temperatures typical of the tropics but condense in the cooler upper latitudes; these characteristics cause them to concentrate near the poles. POPs can now be found virtually everywhere in the world; they are present in the bark of tropical trees, in the blubber of whales in the northern Pacific, in the stratosphere high overhead. POPs are also biologically persistent: they are fat soluble, so they tend to bioaccumulate in the tissues of living things. Bioaccumulation is an ecological process of concentration. The offending chemical tends to become more and more concentrated as it moves up the food chain: shrimp with low-level PCB contamination, for example, will mean shrimp-eating fish with higher levels of contamination, and fish-eating eagles with even higher levels. Of course, the process can include humans as well. Take dioxins, the notorious group of chemical byproducts that contains several potent carcinogens. It has been estimated that 90 percent of the dioxins that contaminate people come not from direct exposure, but from the consumption of animal products—fish, red meat, even ice cream. It's thought that nearly all people on earth are contaminated to some degree by POPs.[8]

"O" as in organic: POPs are carbon-based compounds.

All but the simplest organic compounds—the chemical class that contains not just POPs but proteins, carbohydrates, and many other substances as well—are built from a chain or ring of carbon atoms. Hydrogen and oxygen atoms are generally arrayed along this carbon backbone, and the structure may contain other elements as well. POPs are likely to have at least one element other than these three; in the known POPs, it's generally chlorine. (Chlorine's role is discussed below.) It's helpful to note that not all manufactured chemicals are organic; inorganic chemicals play key industrial roles as well. Sulfuric acid (H_2SO_4), for example, is a key feedstock for much chemical production, especially fertilizer. But most commercially important inorganics, like sulfuric acid, aren't synthetic in the sense of being completely artificial—they occur in nature. And synthetic or not, only around 100,000 inorganic chemicals are known. Contrast that with the many millions of organic compounds now known—most of them wholly artificial—and you can begin to get an idea of the stupifying variety in molecular structure that carbon permits.[9]

"P" as in pollutant: POPs are highly toxic.

Because they bioaccumulate, POPs can cause long-term health effects. This type of toxicity is known as *chronic toxicity*. (If a compound inflicts serious injury immediately after exposure, it is said to have a high *acute toxicity*; in the quantities in which they are usually encountered, POPs are generally less poisonous in this sense.) The mechanisms that underlie toxicity in POPs are not well understood, but a range of processes is clearly involved. For example, some POPs are thought to be hormonally active compounds that mimic natural chemical messengers and throw the body's endocrine system into disarray. Others are carcinogens; still others interfere with fetal development, and so on. One of the reasons that POPs are so difficult to deal with is that they can inflict this kind of damage long after exposure and at extremely low doses. For example, one of the dioxins, TCDD, may disrupt the reproductive capabilities of an animal or the normal intellectual development of a child in the parts per *trillion* range. According to the World Health Organization (WHO), a person who weighs 80 kilograms (176 pounds) shouldn't be exposed to more than 320 trillionths of a gram of TCDD per day.[10]

In sum, POPs are stable organic compounds whose longevity allows them to be widely dispersed in the environment. They are fat soluble, which allows them to accumulate in the bodies of living things. And they generally have a relatively low acute toxicity but a high chronic toxicity, which can express itself in a variety of dysfunctions.

As you can see from this description, chemicals are classed as POPs on the basis of their behavior rather than their structure (apart from the fact that they must be organic). Theoretically, an organic chemical of any form could be a POP, but certain structural features are strongly associated with the basic POP characteristics. For example, there is a class of organic compounds called aromatic hydrocarbons, whose molecules have a carbon backbone that includes a ring structure. A classic example is benzene. Often these molecules have several carbon rings, in which case they are called polycyclic aromatic hydrocarbons, or PAHs. PAHs tend to be stable and fat soluble. If you take one of these molecules and attach an atom from the halogen group of elements (chlorine or bromine, for example), you will probably make it even more stable and fat soluble. In some cases, you will also make it quite toxic. If you've invented a new halogenated PAH, you have an excellent candidate POP on your hands. Most well-known POPs fall into this category; all of the "dirty dozen" chemicals belong in it.[11]

Of the elements in the halogen group, one in particular has been used extensively by the chemical industry: chlorine. Organic compounds containing chlorine, known as organochlorines, do not normally occur in large quantities in nature. (There are a few exceptions, such as salt marsh emissions of methyl chloride.) In the chemical economy, however, organochlorines are a key component. There is no single chemical virtue that chlorine imparts to a synthetic molecule—its value to chemists might best be described as an expansion of options. Chlorine will snap firmly into place along an organic molecule's carbon backbone, and it can be used to anchor all sorts of interesting structures. Such structures might make a chemical more toxic—an advantage if you're designing a pesticide. They might alter the chemical's solubility—an important consideration for solvents, plasticizers, and so on. They might make the chemical more reactive or conversely, more persistent. Such possibilities go some way towards explaining why there are around 11,000 organochlorines in commerce, including various pesticides, solvents, plastics, pharmaceuticals, and many other products. Chlorine has become, in the words of W. Joseph Stearns, former Director of Chlorine Issues for the Dow Chemical Company, "the single most important ingredient in modern [industrial] chemistry." It has also become one of the most suspect: most known POPs are organochlorines. In addition to being PAHs, all the "dirty dozen" chemicals fall into this category as well. (The relationships between these various categories are shown in Figure 1.)[12]

So many dangerous chemicals in so few groups: clearly, this situation raises a couple of basic questions. To take the narrower issue first: are organochlorines inherently more likely to be POPs than organobromines, say, or other organohalogens? Is chlorine, in other words, the most dangerous halogen? The answer, it would seem, is not necessarily—our problems with chlorine are largely a result of the fact that it is the halogen that we have used most extensively. The toxicology of the other halogens is not as well understood. But as the liabilities of many organochlorines have become clearer, chemists have increasingly turned to the other halogens in the hope of synthesizing chemicals with similar useful properties but with lower toxicity. Similar virtues, however, often seem to mean similar vices. Thus, for example, the polybrominated flame retardants developed as substitutes for PCBs have themselves proved to be persistent and bioaccumulative. Bromine is not necessarily a "kinder" element than chlorine.[13]

Then there's the broader issue concerning halogens in general: do most of the long-term risks created by the modern chemical economy fall within this group? The answer would appear to be the same: not necessarily. The risks follow the commerce, and the industry is already producing some nonhalogenated POPs—for example, certain organometals used in marine paints. Innovation in other chemical groups could presumably create other types of POPs as well.[14]

It's also important to understand that long-term risks

FIGURE 1

Where POPs Fit in the Commercial Chemical Universe

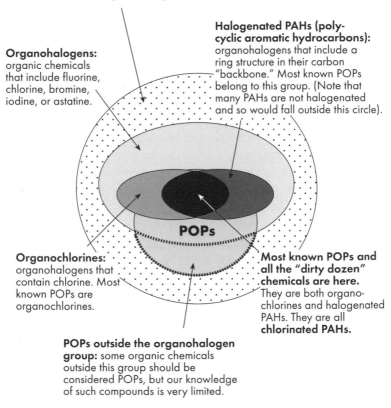

Organic chemicals: compounds that contain carbon. Organic chemicals are the basis of life—carbohydrates, for example, and proteins belong to this class. Organics are also the basis for the synthetic chemical industry; there are probably between 50,000 and 100,000 synthetic organic chemicals in commerce.

Halogenated PAHs (polycyclic aromatic hydrocarbons): organohalogens that include a ring structure in their carbon "backbone." Most known POPs belong to this group. (Note that many PAHs are not halogenated and so would fall outside this circle).

Organohalogens: organic chemicals that include fluorine, chlorine, bromine, iodine, or astatine.

Organochlorines: organohalogens that contain chlorine. Most known POPs are organochlorines.

Most known POPs and all the "dirty dozen" chemicals are here. They are both organochlorines and halogenated PAHs. They are all chlorinated PAHs.

POPs outside the organohalogen group: some organic chemicals outside this group should be considered POPs, but our knowledge of such compounds is very limited.

Note: Circles are not drawn to scale.

are not created solely by POPs. Depending on the circumstances of their production and use, other chemicals may create long-term problems, even if they do not come within the POPs definition. Organochlorine solvents, for example, are generally not persistent enough to qualify as POPs, yet many of them are quite toxic: they have been linked to miscarriages, infertility, kidney and liver cancer, and various immune system disorders. Some of these chemicals are very common industrial materials. TCE (trichloroethylene), for instance, is widely used for degreasing metal; perc (perchloroethylene) is the standard drycleaning solvent. And while such chemicals may not be persistent, they may degrade into other toxic substances that are much more stable. Among the breakdown products of both TCE and perc, for example, are potent plant and animal toxins. Despite their lack of persistence, TCE and perc are relevant to the POPs debate because of their toxicity and ubiquity. Some chlorinated solvents are now effectively considered POPs by certain regional agreements, notably the 1992 OSPAR Convention for the Protection of the Marine Environment of the Northeast Atlantic.[15]

This situation conjures up a basic philosophical problem—a problem at the heart of the modern chemical economy. Very likely, a substantial proportion of the synthetics now in commerce pose no greater risk than many other phenomena that we readily tolerate. Even among the organochlorines, there may be thousands of chemicals that could be assigned to this "acceptable risk" category. But the chemical industry is continually introducing additional chemicals, and of course, it's continuing to pump out more and more of the chemicals already in production. (Even chemicals with very bad records do not necessarily go out of production entirely; they often continue to be produced and used in countries where regulations are lax.)

In general, regulators have responded to this situation by developing standardized tests for new compounds, although the thoroughness of these tests varies greatly, depending on the country and the use to which the com-

pound will be put (pesticides, for example, are normally tested more thoroughly than solvents). The tests may be upgrad-
ed periodically, as the toxicology improves, and the
improved tests may then be applied to chemicals already in
commerce. But this can be an extremely cumbersome
process. In 1996, for example, the United States launched a
major pesticide reevaluation program, in the light of new
research on how these chemicals can affect children, whose
rapid metabolism and rapid rate of physical development
make them more vulnerable to certain kinds of toxins. By
1999, screening had been completed on less than half of pesticide "registrations." (The United States regulates pesticides
by designating specific uses permitted for each chemical;
each such use is known as a registration.)[16]

Such efforts tend to bog down, not just because of the
number of chemicals involved, but because of a kind of testing paradox: the more sophisticated a test becomes, the
more complex and expensive it tends to be. And the
advances in toxicology raise an even more fundamental
issue: what are the current tests missing? Endocrine disruption, for example, wasn't a concern just a decade ago. Who
knows what we'll be testing for in another decade? And
beyond the testing of individual chemicals, there looms the
problem of testing for the overlapping effects of *several chemicals*—a phenomenon about which we know very little.[17]

So this is the philosophical problem: there is a mis-
match between the chemically innovative industry and the
essentially reactive posture of the agencies charged with regulating it. The agencies have no realistic hope of "catching
up" with the industry, and the gap between the two would
not appear to favor human and environmental health over
the long term. What is needed is fundamental reform—a
change that goes far deeper than conventional regulation.
That reform could start with a very simple but revolutionary
idea: it's wise to avoid unnecessary risk. This is the kernel of
one of the environmental movement's core concepts: the
precautionary principle. The principle states that even in the
face of scientific uncertainty, the prudent stance is to restrict

or even prohibit an activity that may cause long-term or irreversible harm.[18]

The principle reverses the usual burden of proof. In most environmental controversies today, that burden usually rests with those who are arguing that an activity is dangerous. Such people are usually in the position of having to prove that the risks entailed by the activity are unreasonably high. But we rarely understand environmental risks until after the damage is done—and maybe not even then. That's the problem the principle is meant to address. It shifts the burden of proof from the opponents of the activity to the advocates. It asks them to prove that the risks *aren't* unreasonable. In effect, the principle is a kind of insurance policy against our own ignorance.[19]

In terms of our adoption of new chemicals, a reasonable application of the precautionary principle would require us to assume that for certain chemical classes—organohalogens, for example—any novel compound is potentially dangerous. The next step would be to ask: do we really need it? This kind of inquiry would tend to foster a different kind of innovation, both within the chemical industry and within society as a whole. The emphasis would tend to shift from inventing new chemicals, to inventing new uses for chemicals known to be reasonably safe, and to inventing new procedures that may not be dependent on chemicals at all. Fewer new chemicals would come into commerce; a growing number of established ones would come out. In each of the three industries surveyed below, the basis for this type of innovative shift has already emerged.

Pulp and Paper: Designing the Toxic Out of the System

Paper rivals plastic in its pervasiveness. It's the substance that holds us together intellectually and socially, in the form of books, newspapers, and magazines. It's also perhaps the most common packaging material—48 percent of world paper production is used in this way. And then of course there are "hygenic papers," to use the standard euphemism, and all sorts of specialty papers, for filtering everything from coffee to laboratory chemicals.[20]

Paper has been produced for some 2,000 years, but for most of that time, it was a specialty, artisanal product derived from the fibers of rags and various nonwoody plants including the one from which it gets its name—the giant reed, papyrus. It wasn't until the mid-1800s that paper began to be produced in large quantities from wood fiber, which is how 55 percent of the world's paper is produced today. (Another 38 percent of the total is from recycled fiber, which derives from wood, and 7 percent is from nonwood fibers such as straw.) Worldwide, 294 million tons of paper were produced in 1998, up nearly four-fold from 7.7 million tons in 1961, the first year for which such statistics were collected. (See Figure 2.)[21]

Mass production from woodpulp is the technology that brought paper within the chemical economy. In order to turn wood into papers that are durable and white, the cellulose (wood fiber), must be purified and bleached. The standard bleach has been chlorine, and that has made the pulp and paper sector a major source of POPs and POP-like compounds. In Sweden and the United States, for instance, pulp and paper mills are one of the largest industrial sources of dioxins in water, soil, and paper itself. "When all pathways are considered," writes Joe Thornton, author of *Pandora's Poison*, a recent book on chlorine and POPs, "the bleaching of pulp with chlorine has been and continues to be one of the world's largest sources of persistent organochlorines into the environment." In some regions, pulp and paper is the largest contributor: 90 percent of organochlorines detected in the waters of the Baltic Sea and North American Great Lakes have been traced to pulp mill effluents.[22]

To appreciate the global scale of the problem, it is important to understand what lies behind an ordinary, rather benign-looking sheet of paper. To turn a log into

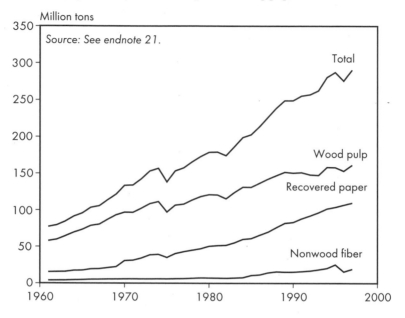

FIGURE 2

World Paper Production, by Fiber Supply, 1961–97

Million tons

Source: See endnote 21.

Total

Wood pulp

Recovered paper

Nonwood fiber

paper, it must first be stripped of its bark and chipped. The chips are then digested into a pulp, a process that releases the cellulose fibers from other materials in the wood, primarily lignin. Lignin is a kind of natural glue—it holds the cellulose fibers together. It typically accounts for one-quarter to one-third of the chemical composition of wood, and the more of it that can be removed, the brighter and more durable the resulting paper will be. Next, the pulp is rinsed and it may be bleached. Finally, it is pressed into paper.[23]

There are basically two ways to make pulp from wood. In mechanical pulping, the chips or sometimes whole logs are heated and forced against metal or stone grinding surfaces. This process captures 90 percent or more of the cellulose but it tends to break the fibers, so the resulting paper is relatively weak. Such low quality pulp is usually destined for newsprint, phone books, and other relatively short-lived products. About 15 percent of world pulp capacity is mechanical.[24]

The other way to produce pulp is through a chemical process in which the chips are cooked in a solution of sulfides. This process captures only about half the cellulose, but it does little appreciable damage to the fibers and it rids them of much more lignin than does mechanical pulping. (It's also responsible for the characteristic rotten egg smell of pulp mills.) Chemical pulp generally produces the highest quality papers. About 42 percent of world pulp capacity is chemical. The remaining capacity (about 43 percent) is in several variants of these two main methods. The most important of these is for handling recycled fiber, which requires very little in the way of chemicals or mechanical processing.[25]

Although any pulp may be bleached, it is primarily the chemical pulps that come in for this treatment. Bleaching whitens the fibers, of course, and it removes residual lignin. It also accounts for virtually all of the industry's organochlorine pollution. At least 40 percent of the world's pulp supply is bleached with chlorine compounds, and until the mid-1990s, the standard method was to use pure, "elemental" chlorine, which produces the largest quantities of toxics.[26]

Industrial scale pulp mills are usually enormous facilities. Such a mill may produce 600 to 1,000 tons of pulp per day; if it is bleaching that pulp with elemental chlorine it will also produce an average of 35 tons of chlorinated byproducts per day. Some 250 different organochlorines have been identified in pulp mill effluent, including several of the "dirty dozen" chemicals—hexachlorobenzene, for instance, and various dioxins and furans. In the United States, the Toxics Release Inventory (a national database of toxic emissions) routinely ranks pulp and paper as the third most polluting of 74 industrial sectors (after chemical producers and the primary metals sector), in terms of emissions per unit of value output.[27]

But it's not just the volume of the emissions and the number of compounds that is troubling—it's also the tendency of these emissions to set off chemical reactions that produce more pernicious compounds. For instance, some initial byproducts, such as chlorolignins, are relatively nontoxic and degrade easily. But they break down into other organochlorines (chlorinated phenols, guaiacols, and cate- chols), some of which tend to be more toxic, more resistant to decomposition, and more likely to bioaccumulate. These compounds, in turn, may form into ones that are even more toxic and long-lived.[28]

As they undergo their chemical metamorphoses, these organochlorines also start their journey into aquatic ecosys- tems, since pulp mills are generally located on rivers, and up the food chain. The potency of some of these chemicals vir- tually guarantees ecological degradation even at minute lev- els. "Fleeting exposure to mere nanograms of dioxin is enough to kill immature fish," according to University of Wisconsin toxicologist Richard Peterson. Even when the chemicals don't kill, they may still have a profound physio- logical and ecological impact. For example, researchers in Florida have linked mill effluent to the "masculinizing" of female fish—in the presence of the effluent, the females developed both behavioral and physical male traits. A study in the late 1980s by the U.S. Environmental Protection Agency (EPA) found high levels of dioxins and furans in fish downstream from pulp mills in sites across the country. Not surprisingly, the states generally ban consumption of fish from rivers and streams in the vicinity of pulp mills. Some of these bans have become a quasi-permanent legal fixture—this is true in parts of the Great Lakes basin, for example.[29]

But even where people aren't consuming the fish, other creatures certainly are, and they are feeling the effects of the poisons. A study of great blue herons near a British Columbia mill, for example, found that the chicks showed stunted growth and usually died before reaching sexual maturity. In similar fashion, otters, mink, eagles, gulls and other fish-eat- ing birds in Canada, the United States, and the Nordic coun- tries have suffered from a variety of reproductive and development disorders. This pattern is typical of bioaccumu- lation: the predator is more vulnerable than its prey. And because top predator populations tend to be relatively small and widely distributed to begin with, this kind of ecological degradation is not likely to be obvious to the casual observer. To anyone but a field biologist, the landscape in question may look reasonably "normal."[30]

This type of ecological degradation can also be a kind of social degradation. In North America as elsewhere, indigenous fishing cultures have been injured by the mills. This has been the fate of Canadian aboriginal people living in eastern Alberta, for example, and U.S. aboriginal people in eastern Maine.[31]

But at least the mills in the industrial world have effluent treatment systems, which capture much of the pollution. Elsewhere, the picture is often very different. There are thousands of small mills using obsolete technologies in China, Brazil, India, and other developing countries. Such mills may not treat their effluent at all—they often simply release it directly into the local waters. Ricardo Carrere and Larry Lohmann note in their book, *Pulping the South*, that millions of small-scale fishers in places as diverse as Kenya and northern Sumatra are losing their livelihoods because of enormous pulp mills spewing forth "some of the most toxic effluent any industry can produce."[32]

The pulp sectors of the developing world usually show a much higher level of emissions per unit of product than their counterparts in North America and western Europe. Less than a quarter of the world's pulp capacity—the sectors of Russia, eastern Europe, Latin America, and Asia excluding Japan—is responsible for about 75 percent of suspended solids emissions, and about 38 percent of organochlorine emissions. (See Table 2.) Although we lack the field studies to prove it, it's a safe bet that the terrain in these areas has also been disproportionately poisoned.[33]

In general, if not necessarily in every region, pulp mill pollution is likely to become an increasingly important environmental issue because of the phenomenal growth in world paper production. In part, the global boom is driven by an important regional shift within the paper economy. North America has long been the industry's stronghold, but more and more pulp is being produced by countries in Asia and

TABLE 2

Average Range of Chemical Pulp Mill Effluent by Region

Region	1999 World Chemical Pulp Production	TSS	COD	AOX
	(percent)	(kilograms per ton)		
North America	53	3-6	40-50	2.1-4.3
Europe	24	4-13	38-90	0.5-4.4
Asia	13	5-24	70-150	2.1-6.6
Latin America	8	5-12	50-76	1.1-4.1
Africa	1.5	8-13	45-90	1.1-3.0

Key:

TSS: total suspended solids (fiber, bark, mud, etc.).

COD: chemical oxygen demand (an indicator that covers all organic matter, the decay of which reduces the oxygen content of the water into which it is released).

AOX: adsorbable organohalogens (essentially, organochlorine pollution).

These categories are standard for measuring pulp mill water pollution.

Source: See endnote 33.

Latin America. Over the period 1992 to 1999, Latin American pulp production grew by 31 percent, to 10.6 million tons. Asia's production grew by 20 percent, to 19.8 million tons, from 1992 to 1997, then it slackened in the wake of the Asian economic downturn. (It stood at 18 million tons in 1999, a 9 percent increase from 1992.)[34]

Several important changes within the paper economy in Asia and Latin America are contributing to this shift, primarily growth in domestic demand, low labor costs, and expanding pulp plantation sectors. The integration of world markets is a factor as well; many of the enormous, new mills in these regions are designed primarily to serve export markets. Another major stimulus to growth is effectively built into the size of some of those mills, which can cost as much as $1.5 to $2 billion to build. The huge investments at stake in these operations are a virtual guarantee that substantial efforts will be made to promote demand for their products.[35]

In response to mounting public and legal pressure to clean up its organochlorine pollution, much of the industry is switching from elemental chlorine to a process that uses chlorine derivatives such as chlorine dioxide (ClO_2). This process is known as "elemental chlorine free" bleaching or ECF. It reduces many organochlorine pollutants (although not all of them) and it can radically cut total organochlorine emissions. The effectiveness of the technology varies considerably depending on the engineering of the plant in which it is installed but generally, ECF can reduce organochlorine emissions from an average of 35 tons per day per mill to something on the order of 7 to 10 tons. ECF technology can be installed relatively cheaply in mills that use the older, elemental process. As increasing numbers of old mills get this retrofit and new ECF mills come on line, the technology is spreading rapidly. (See Figure 3.)[36]

ECF clearly is a form of improvement. In the United States, where paper production grew by almost 10 percent between 1992 and 1996, the industry's elemental chlorine consumption declined by 37.5 percent over the same period. Measurable dioxin emissions from pulp and paper mills in North America dropped 96 percent between 1988 and 1994. And in 1997, the U.S. EPA declared ECF the "best available technology" for meeting the clean air and water standards that the agency is charged with enforcing.[37]

But ECF is a kind of "low tar cigarette" approach to the problem of organochlorine pollution. It reduces pollution, but does not address the fundamental problem—the industry's addiction to a substance that it would be better off avoiding in the first place. There is no need to use chlorine at all in the bleaching process. Pulp can be bleached just as well with hydrogen peroxide, oxygen, or ozone. The processes using these materials are known as totally chlorine free

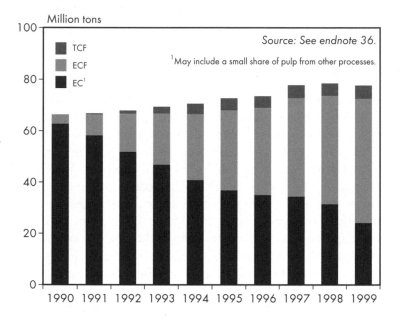

FIGURE 3

World Production of ECF, TCF, and Elemental Chlorine (EC) Pulp, 1990–99

bleaching, or TCF. Obviously, TCF mills produce no organochlorine pollution, except where chlorine residues are present in used paper that the mill is recycling. (Given the current role of chlorine in the paper economy, recycled fiber inevitably contains residual chlorine; papers that were bleached without chlorine but that contain recycled fiber are said to be "process chlorine free." The paper that you are looking at now falls in this category.) And TCF cuts total effluent (including non-organochlorine discharges) by more than half even when measured against the best ECF mills. It releases almost no hazardous air or water pollutants, so the costs of controlling emissions drop substantially. And there's no compromise on the quality of the product: TCF can produce papers that meet or exceed commercial standards for both strength and brightness.[38]

TCF mills are also cheaper to build than either ECF mills or those using elemental chlorine. That's because TCF technology requires less equipment and does not need the special metals necessary for handling chlorine, which is highly corrosive. Its advantages have earned respect from the World Bank, which now gives TCF mill projects more favorable lending rates (although ECF is still the minimum standard). And the technology has proven itself in major installations in various places around the world. In Malaysia, for instance, a joint venture called Malaysia Newsprint Industries opened a huge TCF (process chlorine free) recycled newsprint mill in 1999; the mill is expected eventually to meet three-quarters of that country's newsprint demand. In Scandinavia, TCF accounts for more than a quarter of pulp production. Yet in terms of its global market share, it remains a marginal technology: more than 10 years after it was introduced, only 6 percent of bleached pulp is TCF. (See Figure 3.)[39]

The problem that TCF has encountered is not chemical—it's financial and institutional. TCF is the cheaper option only if the mill in question is being built from scratch. But to convert a present-day facility, ECF is cheaper. To the shareholders and executives of paper companies, ECF may therefore look like a better way of protecting investments—as long as the public can be persuaded to take the "low tar" approach to its paper consumption. And for now, at least, the public appears content. In North America, virtually no TCF pulp is being manufactured (except for some process chlorine free stock). And in Europe, demand for TCF pulp has reportedly declined over the past few years.[40]

Two important lessons can be drawn from this state of affairs. First, the TCF technology is an encouraging real-world confirmation of the precautionary principle. Completely removing a dangerous material from the industrial stream is clearly the best option for overall risk reduction, if that can be done without serious economic disruption and without creating additional environmental or public health risks. TCF appears to pass this test, so in a sense it represents the ideal precautionary scenario. What are the benefits of using chlorine to bleach paper and what are the risks? The risks may not be well defined, but it no longer matters because the benefits have largely evaporated. There are no longer any benefits unique to chlorine bleaching. We can steer clear of the problem entirely.[41]

Avoiding the problem in the first place—this ought to be a basic principle of industrial design. And in paper mill design, the principle can be taken far beyond TCF itself. Even though TCF is not a significant source of chemical pollution, it still imposes some environmental cost, in the form of energy, water, and materials used. So where bleaching is not necessary, it's better to eliminate it outright. United Parcel Service, for example, has eliminated bleached fiber from its packaging material. On a plant level, even greater reductions in environmental cost have been achieved in facilities such as the Louisiana Pacific mill in northern California, where TCF bleaching is combined with a "closed loop" production cycle. These plants are able to recirculate most of their wastewater, thereby reducing water consumption dramatically. Much of the heat in a closed loop system is conserved too; that fact combined with the energy efficiency of the TCF process, allows closed loop plants to greatly reduce their energy consumption as well.[42]

The second lesson is something that any marketing executive can confirm: no product, no matter how good it is, will sell itself. If TCF and "process chlorine free" papers are to become an industry standard, the public will have to buy them. And there is no such thing as spontaneous public demand. The challenge, therefore, is not only to clean up one of the most polluting industries in the world, but to stimulate markets—among the general public, companies, and governments—for paper that is produced in ways that are as clean as the final product looks.

Pesticides: Substituting Knowledge for Synthetics

In 1935, before agriculture was disrupted by World War II, world grain production stood at about 650 million tons. (The major grains account for about half of humanity's food supply, either through direct consumption, or indirectly as livestock feed.) Production would have been much higher, of course, had it not been for the pests—crop diseases, insects, weeds, rodents, and so forth. Pests probably consumed the equivalent of about 30 percent of the harvest.[43]

This year, the grain yield will probably be 1.86 billion tons—nearly a three-fold increase from 1935. Pests will likely claim the equivalent of 37 percent of this harvest, so their share of the agricultural enterprise has increased significantly over the past 65 years. But the most remarkable aspect of their success is that it has come in the face of a massive chemical offensive—an effort that has no precedent in the history of agriculture. To bring in this year's harvest, farmers will apply something on the order of 2.5 million tons of pesticides. The overwhelming share of this material consists of synthetic organic chemicals that did not exist in 1935. Many of these chemicals are several orders of magnitude more toxic than the pesticides available to farmers in the 1930s.[44]

Modern agriculture has a serious chemical dependency—an addiction to pesticides. There is reason to think that this addiction can be broken without prejudice to the harvest. But the cure won't be easy, given the long-established appeal of agriculture's "pesticide paradigm."

In 1939, the Swiss chemist Paul Müller discovered that dichlorodiphenyl trichloroethane (DDT) was an extremely potent pesticide. DDT was apparently first used in 1942 or 1943, as a delousing agent during World War II. In 1948, Müller won a Nobel Prize for his discovery and DDT was being hailed as a sort of chemical miracle. In the minds of its more committed proponents, organic chemistry was on the verge of overcoming one of humanity's oldest scourges: the insects that destroy our crops and infect us with disease.[45]

DDT is toxic to a wide range of insects. In the years following the war, it was rapidly adopted as a general purpose insecticide, first in Europe and North America and then elsewhere. Individual farmers and government agencies applied it for mosquito control, against agricultural pests, against forest pests—against just about every insect that attracted unfavorable attention. This enthusiasm for DDT represented a basic cultural change: large numbers of people had become convinced that it was possible to "solve" pest problems through recourse to extremely toxic chemicals.[46]

DDT was almost immediately followed by other broad spectrum organochlorine pesticides. For example, chlordane was introduced in 1945, just three years after DDT, and it was eventually used not just as an insecticide but as a weed killer. The first widely used organochlorine fungicide, hexachlorobenzene, or HCB, was also introduced in 1945. Heptachlor, a component of chlordane, but four times as toxic, was introduced in its own right in 1948. The same year saw the introduction of toxaphene, which became a favorite for cotton pests and as a livestock dip. During the years 1948 to 1951, three closely related insecticides came on the market: aldrin, dieldrin, and endrin. These compounds have tested as anywhere from five to several hundred times as toxic as DDT, depending upon the type of organism concerned. Their targets included not just insects, but rodents and starlings as well. Finally, 1959 saw the introduction of mirex, which also came to be used as a rodenticide and a fire retardant. Mirex's greatest moment arrived in 1967, when it was used in a 51-million hectare aerial spraying program against the invasive red fire ant (*Solenopsis invicta*), in the U.S. Southeast.[47]

These nine pesticides are all included in the "dirty dozen" list. All of them are quintessential POPs—extremely persistent, bioaccumulative, mobile, and highly toxic. All have been banned or heavily restricted in at least 60 countries, making them relatively easy targets for elimination under the treaty. Most are no longer even in production. The main exception is DDT, which is now banned for agricultural use in at least 86 countries but which is still widely employed for mosquito control. (DDT's role in mosquito control is discussed below.) Small quantities of toxaphene and HCB are also still being manufactured in developing countries, but most HCB is now produced unintentionally, as a byproduct of solvent manufacturing.[48]

Even though these compounds have largely been relegated to the chemical junkyard, they are still very much a part of our world. The cumulative quantity of just six of them is estimated to be more than 7 million tons—and that is probably a gross underestimate, since production data are often unavailable or incomplete. (For endrin, heptachlor, and mirex, the data do not provide an adequate basis for an estimate.) The biological legacy of this chemical use is unclear, but given the potency and longevity of these compounds, it is likely to be considerable. It's also likely to be global, since these pesticides appear to contaminate virtually every ecosystem on the planet. And it's estimated that some 100,000 tons of banned or obsolete pesticides are improperly stored in the developing world; presumably much of this material will eventually leak out into the environment.[49]

Since the mid-1940s, pesticide production has increased by a factor of 42.

One of the most comprehensive records of this form of pollution is the bark of living trees, which scientists can test to map the extent of contamination. The testing of trees at more than 90 temperate and tropical sites worldwide turned up *no sites* that were free from DDT, chlordane, and dieldrin. Humanity itself is subject to a similar level of exposure: DDT remains one of the most commonly detected pesticides in human breast milk samples.[50]

At their advent, the organochlorines had been hailed as a substantial safety improvement over earlier, arsenic-based pesticides, and they might have retained that reputation much longer, had they not become so excessively overused. A full public indictment of organochlorine and many other pesticides did not appear until 1962, with the publication of Rachel Carson's now classic work, *Silent Spring*, but some experts had begun to doubt the wisdom of their use much earlier. Even by 1950, a sufficient number of scientific alarms were going off to trigger hearings in the U.S. Congress; these hearings eventually resulted in regulations on pesticide residues in food.[51]

But regulating on the fringes of the problem did not affect the basic appeal of the pesticide paradigm. The industry response to these initial concerns was essentially to rework the same formula, by producing new pesticides that were meant to be less persistent and bioaccumulative than the original products. For example, despite its current status as a "dirty dozen" chemical, mirex was initially recommended as environmentally benign. Many of these "kinder, gentler" organochlorines are rote variations on established products: methoxychlor and dicofol are close relatives of DDT. But some innovation went farther afield; endosulfan, for instance, includes the element sulfur in its structure. And increasingly, the manufacturers were broadening the range of product applications: in addition to the organochlorine insecticides, a growing line of organochlorine herbicides and fungicides appeared.[52]

Another front of chemical innovation involved the development of organophosphate and carbamate insecticides. (These derive from phosphoric and carbamic acids, respectively.) A few organophosphates had long been known, but like DDT, their pesticidal properties were not described until the late 1930s, when a German scientist, Gerhard Schrader, realized that they were nerve poisons. Some organophosphates were developed as military weapons by Germany; others began a career as pesticides. Among the better known members of this pesticide class are chlorpyrifos, diazinon, malathion, and parathion.[53]

The organophosphates and carbamates are not POPs because, by and large, they aren't very persistent. But they are certainly poisonous to people as well as to insects. They tend to have substantial acute toxicity. Farmworkers subject to chronic exposure may also develop serious neurological problems. Organophosphates have been an enormous economic success: in the United States, they account for about half of all insecticides used. They are found in a vast range of products and are sprayed on most food crops.[54]

But even though they break down too readily to be POPs, organophosphates and carbamates certainly are persistent enough to ride the food supply from farmer to consumer. For example, the U.S.-based Consumers Union, a consumer advocacy group, reports that domestic fruits and vegetables often exceed the safe exposure limit set by the U.S. EPA for young children. And in June 2000, the U.S. National Academy of Sciences estimated that 25 percent of childhood developmental and behavioral problems in the United States are caused by a combination of genetic factors and exposure to neurotoxic chemicals, including lead, PCBs, and organophosphates.[55]

In response to such concerns, the U.S. EPA is re-examining several dozen organophosphates currently on the market and in July 2000, the agency announced plans to cancel several registrations of one of the most commonly used members of this class: chlorpyrifos, the active ingredient in Dursban. Bans of various organophosphates have been enacted in a growing number of other countries as well, including Great Britain, Argentina, Indonesia, and the Philippines.[56]

Currently, probably around 600 different chemicals are used as active ingredients in pesticides. And in terms of aggregate use, the industry has seen enormous expansion since the mid-1940s. The production of active ingredients has escalated roughly 42-fold, from 60,000 tons in 1945 to some 2.5 million tons in 1995. Worldwide, about $31 billion in pesticides is applied by farmers to their crops, by homeowners to their lawns, by maintenance crews to buildings, and by health officials to the areas they are treating for insect-borne disease. As the quantity of pesticide applied has risen, so has its toxicity; the formulations sold today are 10- to 100- times as potent as those marketed in 1975.[57]

Traditionally, about 80 percent of global pesticide use has occurred in industrial countries, but over the past four decades, the spread of pesticide-intensive farming in the developing world has made these chemicals an important export commodity. About 37 percent of production is now traded internationally. (See Figure 4.) Domestic production is also on the rise in the developing world. China, India, and Brazil are among the developing countries planning major new pesticide plants.[58]

The public health and ecological costs of the industry remain poorly defined but there are many reasons for regarding them as substantial. Worldwide, according to WHO, more than 500 people die and another 8,000 are nonfatally poisoned by pesticides every *day*. (Many of the fatalities are farmers who commit suicide because of crop failures.) Recent findings suggest that people chronically exposed to high pesticide levels are more likely to develop heart disease, serious immunodeficiencies, and cancers of the immune system (non-Hodgkin's lymphoma, leukemia, and myeloma).[59]

Nearly 40 years after *Silent Spring*, pesticides continue to do extensive damage to wildlife. Biologists estimate that some 67 million birds fall prey to pesticides each year in the United States alone. Pesticide-induced deformities have been found in many kinds of wild animals—in alligators in the Florida Everglades, eagles in the North American Great Lakes basin, fish in Great Britain, vultures in India. Even when they are not fatal, such deformities are liable to affect the long-term viability of wildlife populations. Organochlorine herbicides are even suspected as a factor in the decline of some European forests.[60]

But perhaps the most remarkable aspect of the pesticide industry is the way it has changed the creatures we are trying to kill. Continual pesticide use introduces what geneticists call a strong "selection pressure" for resistance. That's because no pesticide is 100 percent effective. Some individual pests invariably survive exposure, and with their cousins out of the way, they have plenty of room to breed. If they owe their survival to genetic resistance, then their offspring

FIGURE 4

Pesticide Exports and Imports in Industrial and Developing Countries, 1961–98

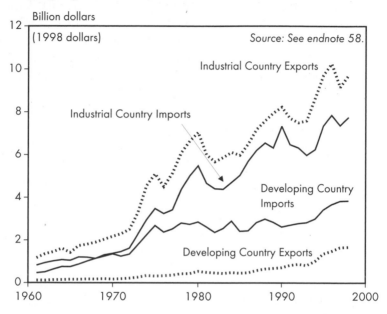

are likely to prosper as well. Soon the whole population may show signs of resistance. Even if there is no genetic resistance initially, it may develop if the survivors are challenged by the chemical year after year. Under such circumstances, any mutation that confers resistance is likely to cause a population explosion.[61]

Resistance to DDT appeared as early as 1946, only one year into the first major public health campaign to use the chemical (an effort to suppress mosquitoes and flies in Italy). Today, pesticide resistance has been detected in about 1,000 major pest species—insects and mites, plant diseases and weeds. And a growing number of these species are resistant to *multiple* pesticides. (See Figure 5.)[62]

But it is possible to interrupt this process, and increasing numbers of farmers are doing it. These people have abandoned the "pesticide treadmill" in favor of farming techniques that use synthetic pesticides only as a last resort, or that avoid them entirely. Integrated Pest Management (IPM) is the general term for agricultural systems that reduce pesticide use by giving preference to non-chemical pest management strategies. Organic agriculture is a more complete development of this approach: it uses no synthetic pesticides or synthetic fertilizers at all. (There is one exception to this rule: it may use some naturally-occurring chemicals that have pesticidal properties.)[63]

As with TCF paper bleaching, the IPM and organic systems are proven technologies. They are backed both by hard scientific data and by real-life farmers. Recently, tens of thousands of rice farmers in China, for example, have demonstrated that a very simple form of polyculture—growing multiple varieties of rice in the same paddies—could double yields without the use of any synthetic chemicals. (The increase was due mainly to reductions in pest losses but partly also to the more efficient nutrient uptake that is typical of polycultural systems.) A U.N. Food and Agriculture Organization study of seven Asian countries found that rice farmers practicing IPM were able to cut their pesticide use by an average of 46 percent, while boosting yields, on average, by 10 percent. In the U.S. Midwest, farmers who produce grain and soybean organically are finding that their net profits equal or surpass those from conventional production, even when they do not charge the premium prices that organic crops generally command. Organic systems are viable in the marketplace not just because they are highly productive, but also because pesticides are very expensive: when farmers go organic, they typically see a huge drop in their production costs.[64]

It is possible to mass produce food and fiber with very low levels of synthetic pesticides, and perhaps with none at all. But the fact that it's possible doesn't mean that it's easy; on the contrary, IPM and organic agriculture require considerable skill. Skill is the basis of an emerging alternative agricultural paradigm, which seeks to substitute farmers' labor and knowledge for reliance on synthetic chemicals.

FIGURE 5

Global Count of Pesticide Resistant Species, 1908–98

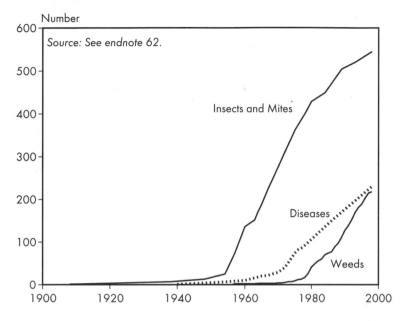

There is a vast fund of knowledge to draw upon in developing such methods. Agriculture is roughly 10 millennia old. Previous generations of farmers have built an intimate and encyclopediac understanding of crop, field, and pest—an understanding that survives in traditional agricultural practices all over the world, and that modern agronomists, in various ways, are struggling to preserve. A full account of these practices is obviously beyond the scope of any single work, but if they were to be reduced to a few general, interrelated principles, they might look something like this.

Grow diversity. In conventional agriculture, breeding and production are separate operations, but in traditional agriculture, they are integrated. The genetic resource is right out in the field—not purchased in seed packets from a company. And the farmer's job is not just to bring in the harvest, but to maintain and enrich this genetic treasure. This is done mainly by cultivating many different forms of a crop, and by careful selection of the seed that will be used for replanting in the next year.

Polyculture offers another major advantage as well. It's a safety net against crop failure, since no single stress— whether a pest, drought, or unseasonable frost—is likely to be able to overwhelm every variety in the field. And when the stress is a pest, there's an automatic dampening effect, since a pest's favorite variety is likely to be intermingled with many other, less favored ones. Polycultures often involve more than just multiple varieties of a single crop—they may include several crops in the same field. Such schemes make for a very efficient use of soil nutrients, and they further reduce pest losses.

Adapt the farming to the site—not the other way around. Conventional agriculture is essentially imposed on a site, in the form of an artificial system that consists of a particular crop variety and interlocking synthetic inputs. The result is generally a dense, chemically dependent monoculture that tends to pollute surrounding ecosystems with pesticide and fertilizer run-off. Traditional agriculture, on the other hand, works with the local ecological processes. For example, farmers often "invite" the local wild flora back into the farmscape, by planting hedgerows and woodlots, by tolerating a certain amount of "weediness," and by allowing fields to go fallow occasionally. The results sometimes look unkempt but they are actually extremely efficient. The wild flora yield additional goods—fruit, for instance, or medicines, or firewood. They help control pests by providing habitat for pest predators, like insectivorous birds. They prevent erosion, restore soil quality, and conserve water. The crucial difference here is continuity: traditional farming certainly changes landscapes, but it doesn't take a *tabula rasa* approach to the process.

Know your friends and enemies. Conventional agriculture is essentially prescriptive; in large measure, its techniques are contained in the instructions that come with the seed, fertilizer, and pesticide that it uses. It's true that traditional agriculture is generally very conservative—traditional farmers are often skeptical of new crops or new growing techniques. But within their cultural context, such farmers generally have an extensive fund of useful knowledge upon which they can draw as they see fit. For example, they may know about plants that can be used to discourage certain pests, about how to use livestock and fire to maintain certain types of planting systems, about nitrogen-fixing "green manure" crops, and so forth. Within the traditional system, the farmer is a sort of "free agent."[65]

Essentially, IPM and organic agriculture draw upon these traditional farming elements, but add two ideas specifically about pest management. First, the most effective pest management is preventive: healthy soil and healthy crops generally have fewer pest problems. And second, when faced with a pest problem, one should adopt a graduated approach that starts with the least toxic treatment and moves to progressively more toxic treatments if satisfactory results are not obtained.

IPM and organic techniques themselves are often extensions of traditional practices. For instance, the "active ingredients" in some plants that have traditionally been used to fend off pests are now in commercial production as pesticides, or they are being used as models for the synthesis of analogous compounds. Synthetic pyrethrins, for example, are modeled on natural insecticides found in some chrysanthemum species. There are however, several drawbacks with this approach. Dependency even on these relatively benign pesticides risks a return to the "pesticide treadmill." And there is controversy over the legitimacy of patenting such substances.[66]

Less controversial is the practice of intercropping with plants that can suppress pests, another traditional practice that is winning wider recognition. For example, several members of the cabbage and mustard genus (*Brassica*) can be used in this fashion. This approach can be extended to other types of organisms as well. For instance, predatory insects, such as ladybugs or lacewings, can be effective pest control agents. (It's important, however, to avoid releasing invasive organisms—in such cases the remedy may well be worse than the disease.)[67]

IPM and organic agriculture may also incorporate technical innovations that have no exact traditional analog. Some growers, for instance, use synthetic pheromones (chemicals that insects release to attract mates) to disrupt reproduction in pest moth species. Pheromone bait confuses the male moths so they do not mate as frequently, which helps keep the pest population low. Pheromones are species-specific; that's a huge ecological advantage, because nonpest insects aren't injured. And resistance to pheromones is unlikely to develop, because they are chemicals that the pest itself manufactures and uses. Some researchers hope to extend this approach by isolating various chemicals that certain plants produce to discourage the insects that attack them.[68]

One of the most promising aspects of IPM and organic agriculture is their potential as a tool for development. In Vietnam, for example, almost half of the country's farmers have now been trained in basic IPM techniques. Most of them live in the rice-growing regions of the South, where they have reduced their use of pesticides and increased profits. Agriculture officials hope to expand the training northward, where agriculture is increasingly becoming mechanized. In Uganda, farmers have been working with government officials and NGOs since 1994, to develop organic cotton farming methods. More than 7,000 farmers in this central African nation now supply about 10 percent of the world's organic cotton. On average, their farms are more productive than conventional Ugandan cotton farms. Organically grown cotton from Uganda is now reaching the shelves of Gap clothing stores in Europe.[69]

It is difficult to gauge the global extent of IPM because so many different farming practices lay claim to that title. But organic agriculture is better defined, and it is clearly booming, thanks to a mix of independent certification standards, government subsidies, and favorable returns. Worldwide, more than 7 million hectares—an area about the size of South Carolina—are now producing organic food and fiber. Much of this area is in North America and Australia, although a larger percentage of farmland is organic in Europe: 0.2 percent of cropland is now certified organic in the United States, compared to nearly 10 percent in several European nations, where subsidies favor the switch to organic. Although their overall contribution is still small, developing countries account for an increasing share of organic production. Currently, for example, just 0.01 percent of China's farmland (470,000 hectares) is dedicated to "Green Food," the country's organic equivalent. But over the next decade, Chinese officials predict organic food will supply 1 percent of this nation's food needs. (The rice polyculture tests, while not organic, suggest that China's potential is far greater than this.)[70]

Organic farming is the fastest growing sector in agriculture.

The financial statistics are considerably more impressive than the cropland numbers. Globally, consumers now spend $22 billion a year on organic products. Organic farming is the fastest growing sector in the agricultural economy. In the United States, which accounts for about a quarter of the market, trade has been growing by nearly 25 percent annually over the last decade. Nearly half of the major U.S. supermarkets now carry organic products. In Japan, demand is growing by more than 20 percent a year. Companies from McDonald's to Patagonia now buy at least some organic ingredients.[71]

The market is hardly limited to rich countries. Farmers in 130 countries now produce organically grown food. In many parts of the world, people are now willing to pay higher prices for organically produced crops, which typically cost about 20 percent more than conventional crops. Brazil hosts organic farmers' markets; there are supermarkets in Argentina offering organic produce, and people in Malaysia and India are buying organic. In many developing countries, there is increasing interest not just in domestic markets, but in export possibilities as well. Already, according to UNCTAD, the U.N. agency that monitors international trade, organic food is "a major business on the global market."[72]

But there is another form of pesticide use, beyond agriculture, which may pose an even greater challenge to our ability to manage pests safely. All the ecological, political, and social complexities of pest management, it seems, come into play in humanity's relationship with the nearly 60 mosquitoes in the genus *Anopheles*, the carriers of malaria. Malaria is the reason that it is so difficult to let go of DDT. Although malaria is not often in the news, it is one of the most serious problems that humanity faces. Some 40 percent of the world's population lives in areas where malaria is prevalent. Each year, nearly half a billion people become sick and at least 1 million people are killed by malaria, primarily in sub-Saharan Africa. (The mortality data are probably a gross underestimate since most deaths occur at home and are never formally registered.) Malaria exacts an especially heavy toll among infants and young children: about four children under the age of five succumb every *minute*.[73]

There are many reasons for the disease's continued grip on humanity. Public health services are lacking in many regions, and the disease organism, the *Plasmodium* parasite, has developed resistance to most of the drugs aimed at it— just as insects develop resistance to insecticides. Because of this drug resistance, and because *Anopheles* mosquitoes are widely distributed within the humid tropics, mosquito control is essential to malaria control. The mosquito populations are carrying an immense reservoir of the parasite.[74]

Since 1955, WHO has had a standard recommendation for *Anopheles* control: heavy reliance on DDT. Many doctors and public health officials still argue that DDT remains the best weapon, particularly where other options are too expensive, or when alternative pesticides fail to stem the mosquitoes, as happened in recent years in KwaZulu Natal.[75]

While there is no doubt that malaria is far more deadly than DDT, the growing arsenal of alternatives and the lack of progress against the disease now call into question the use of

DDT as a first resort. Not surprisingly, there are now numerous dissenters from the DDT approach among the ranks of the doctors and public health officials fighting malaria. And even WHO has shifted its policy somewhat. In 1993, it issued new recommendations, which sanctioned the spraying of DDT indoors only, and recognized the importance of safer insecticides. More recently, WHO's Expert Committee on Malaria announced that DDT "should only be used in well defined, high or special risk situations." In late 1998, WHO, the World Bank, and several other international institutions launched a "Roll Back Malaria" campaign, which employs the latest malaria fighting tools, both chemical and non-chemical. The campaign allows for highly controlled use of DDT in emergencies, but its focus is on strengthening public health systems generally.[76]

No single method of fighting the disease will work in every region where it occurs. But malaria control—and indeed, the control of many other vector-borne diseases—has developed public health versions of some basic IPM principles. This approach even has an analogous name: IVM, or Integrated Vector Management. (See Table 3.) Here are three overlapping principles:[77]

Use the least toxic option first. Mosquito control is no longer just a matter of spraying insecticides. It involves education about how to reduce mosquito habitat around the home. It includes simple, nonpesticidal control methods, such as installing window screens to keep mosquitoes from biting at night, draining unnecessary standing water, or covering the surface of open latrines to prevent mosquitoes from breeding.[78]

And certainly, it will continue to involve the use of pesticides, but not necessarily DDT. Researchers in sub-Saharan Africa have demonstrated that bednets soaked in synthetic pyrethrins can reduce the transmission of malaria by 30 to 60 percent and childhood mortality by up to 30 percent. If used in combination with other control and treatment strategies, these bednets might prevent half of all deaths from malaria. They could be easily introduced at the local

TABLE 3

Integrated Pest Management and Integrated Vector Management: Selected Parallels

Management Option	IPM	IVM	Environmental and Health Risks
General	Diversify the system. Use polyculture, more complex crop rotations, and regular fallow periods.	Reduce vector habitat. With mosquitoes, the emphasis should probably be on draining unneeded standing water or covering it.	Very low, as long as natural bodies of water are not drained.
Physical barriers and traps	Where feasible, use netting over crops, weedblocking fabric over soil, and insect traps.	Use bed nets, window and door screens, and baited traps to reduce vector presence indoors.	Very low, except where pesticides are used in the bed nets or traps.
Biological control	Release predatory insects, such as lacewings, preying mantises, or ladybugs to keep plant-eating insects in check.	Release of various mosquito predators, especially mosquito-eating fish, has been a common mosquito control technique.	Moderate to high because of the danger of causing bioinvasions. The introduction of mosquito-eating fish, in particular, has been ecologically disruptive in many areas.
Pesticides	Use pesticides only as a last resort. The least toxic chemicals should take precedence over more toxic ones. "Natural pesticides" are usually preferred. All pesticides should be targeted and resistance should be monitored.	As with IPM.	High. Even the use of "alternative pesticides" may have serious health and environmental effects. And resistance is virtually inevitable if such use becomes routine.

Source: See endnote 77.

level and are relatively cost effective: $10 for a bednet plus $1 for a year's supply of insecticide. Over the next five years, Roll Back Malaria is planning a thirty-fold increase in the use of bednets in Africa. Of course, alternative insecticides can still cause health problems and they can certainly trigger resistance. (Resistance to some pyrethrins is already spreading rapidly in Africa.) Limiting the agricultural use of some alternative pesticides may help preserve their utility against mosquitoes.[79]

IPM and mosquito control also converge on this principle: *know the local terrain*. The world's malaria zones vary enormously, and the best option in one region may not be a good idea in another. Of course, knowledge of place is not just physical and ecological—it's also social. Finding ways to build community support is just as important as finding the mosquitoes themselves.

Finally, the principle that public health officials are perhaps the farthest from realizing: *know your enemy*. The malaria parasite is still in many respects a mysterious organism, as can be seen from our failure thus far to devise a vaccine for it. The Bill and Melinda Gates Foundation recently created a $50 million fund for malaria vaccine research, which may help catalyze innovation. One promising prototype involves a kind of genetically engineered protein that attacks four stages of the parasite's lifecycle. (The usual approach is to focus on a single stage.)[80]

But perhaps the biggest single unmet need, as far as this principle is concerned, is the study of the mosquito vectors. Given their accessibility and their unfortunate importance to humanity, it's amazing how little we know about them— about their mating interactions, for example, their population dynamics, or their food sources other than human blood. Ellis McKenzie, a Harvard biologist, was quoted recently in the *New Scientist* about this matter: "Our ignorance of the basic biology of *Anopheles gambiae* [the principal African vector] seems nearly encyclopediac."[81]

Our ignorance of the parasite and its vector is probably blocking progress on many fronts. Given the lack of progress, a commitment to abandoning DDT might seem unrealistic. But this situation may not differ fundamentally from the situation with dioxins and furans, for example. These materials are the byproducts of a wide range of industrial processes, and their complete elimination is probably beyond our current technical capabilities. But agreeing in principle to eliminate them would still be a very useful political act, because it would build demand for the technologies that could eventually make that goal a reality. The same strategy should be applied to DDT: substantial reductions are possible immediately under the IVM approach. Elimination could eventually follow if a broad political mandate is built for that goal. But given the nature of our dependence on DDT, this mandate will also have to aim at malaria control.

As with TCF paper making, alternative forms of pest management suggest a couple of conclusions that may have broad relevance for the reform of the chemical economy. First, it's sometimes best to substitute a practice for a product: organic growing practices, for example, may make more sense than pesticide products. It's true that products usually have greater "charisma" than practices. It's easy to get into the habit of thinking that buying the right product is the way to solve a problem, or at least the way to make substantial progress against it. But as humanity's relationship with pests demonstrates, there may be no "right product." There may be only a set of highly dynamic relationships, which must be managed indefinitely. And as every effective manager knows, tools are useful, but what really counts is skill.

Second, reform can be strengthened by engaging more than a single objective at once. Looking for "overlapping" objectives can help build a broader mandate for change. Eliminating DDT, for example, is not just about reducing exposure to a toxic pesticide—it's about reducing exposure to malaria as well. Curing agriculture's addiction to poisonous chemicals is not just a way of ensuring a healthier food supply—it's also a way of restoring ecological integrity to agricultural systems. It may be helpful to assume that every major objective has several potential constituencies. Making change happen may be primarily a matter of putting all the relevant constituencies together.

PVC: Turning Complex Problems into Multiple Opportunities

In terms of production volume, PVC, or polyvinylchloride, is the second most common plastic in the world after poly-ethylene. But in terms of its spectrum of applications, PVC is second to none. Polyethylene is used primarily in medical devices, packaging, electrical insulation, flooring, and some auto components. PVC is put to all these uses as well, and countless others. Currently about 60 percent of PVC production is destined for the construction industry, where it is used for everything from water pipes to siding. Most of the remaining 40 percent is in consumer goods: your phone cord, the dashboard of your car, your credit cards and shower curtain, even the wrap on your sandwich—if you're looking at plastic, there's a good chance that you're looking at PVC.[82]

First manufactured in 1936, PVC is now being produced at the rate of 22 to 30 million tons per year. (See Figure 6.) Overall, production is accelerating: in the early 1990s, it was growing at the rate of about 2 percent per year; in the first half of this decade, the annual rate of production will likely be more than twice as fast. By 2005, global PVC demand is projected to reach 33 million tons. Quite simply, PVC is now one of the most common synthetic materials in the world. There are few if any major economic activities that it does not touch in one way or another.[83]

Nearly half of the near-term growth in production is expected to occur in Asia, where the industry has prospered despite the 1997-1998 economic crisis. PVC production in Japan, South Korea, and Taiwan increased 21 percent between 1995 and 1999. China's imports of PVC jumped 360

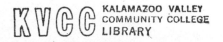

FIGURE 6

PVC Consumption by Region, 1991–2001 (estimated); and PVC Production Capacity, Regional Percentages, 1999

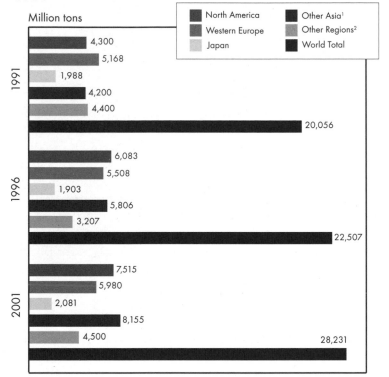

Million tons

Legend:
- North America
- Western Europe
- Japan
- Other Asia[1]
- Other Regions[2]
- World Total

1991
- 4,300
- 5,168
- 1,988
- 4,200
- 4,400
- 20,056

1996
- 6,083
- 5,508
- 1,903
- 5,806
- 3,207
- 22,507

2001
- 7,515
- 5,980
- 2,081
- 8,155
- 4,500
- 28,231

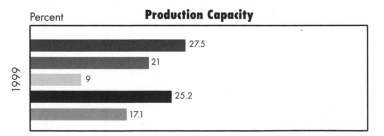

Percent   **Production Capacity**

1999
- 27.5
- 21
- 9
- 25.2
- 17.1

[1]"Other Asia" includes China, Hong Kong, India, Indonesia, Malaysia, Philippines, Singapore, South Korea, Taiwan, and Thailand.

[2]"Other Regions" includes Africa, Eastern Europe, Latin America, Middle East, and Oceania. *Source: See endnote 83.*

percent between 1994 and 1999—a trend that is likely to continue. The primary driver of Asian demand is the construction industry, especially in the region's major cities, such as Beijing, Bangkok, and Manila.[84]

PVC manufacturers are already well placed to serve this market. About 150 companies in 50 different countries currently produce the material, but the largest manufacturers are in Asia. The biggest of all is Japan's Shin-Etsu Chemical Company; Formosa Plastics of Taiwan is the world's number two producer. Manufacturers in South Korea, the United States, and Europe round out the world's top 10 PVC manufacturers, which together accounted for more than 40 percent of global capacity in 1997.[85]

The world's current cumulative burden of PVC probably comes to about 400 million tons. Around 250 million tons of this quantity is most likely in use; the remainder is piling up in landfills, feeding incinerators and backyard fires, or clogging up the recycling stream.[86]

PVC is certainly persistent but it's not a POP. In its pure form, PVC resin appears to be biologically inert. There is no evidence that it bioaccumulates or that it is mobile in the environment, for instance by being susceptible to long range atmospheric transport. But in the full context of its lifecycle, PVC presents a very different picture. Every stage of that lifecycle—from manufacture, to use, to disposal—creates dangerous chemicals, including some of the most notorious POPs.[87]

PVC is the only major commercial plastic that contains chlorine. The other major plastics are almost entirely petroleum-based, but PVC has a chlorine content of up to 45 percent by weight. The high chlorine content can give PVC an economic advantage over other plastics: it helps insulate PVC prices from oil market fluctuations. But chlorine is also PVC's biggest ecological liability.[88]

Chlorine is introduced into the PVC lifecycle at the beginning of the manufacturing process. Basically, it takes three steps to produce PVC resin, and the first of these combines ethylene gas with either elemental chlorine or hydrogen chloride to produce ethylene dichloride, or EDC.

Because of its role in PVC manufacturing, more EDC is produced than most other organic synthetics. In 1997, global
manufacturing capacity for this material stood at 33.5 million tons, a total that is expected to increase in the next few
years. EDC is not persistent, so it isn't a POP. It is, however,
extremely dangerous. According to the hazard ranking system of the U.S.-based NGO Environmental Defense, it ranks
among the top 10 percent of all synthetics, in terms of its
capacity to damage ecological and human health. It's a
known carcinogen and a suspected nerve poison. It may
cause birth defects, and damage the sex organs, heart, lungs,
liver, kidneys, and skin.[89]

For each ton of EDC produced, about 4 kilograms of
byproducts are created. About half of this material consists of
"light ends"—that is, substances that are more volatile than
EDC. These are typically reprocessed into the solvent perchloroethylene. The remaining byproducts are tar-like
"heavy ends," which are simply waste and may end up in the
air, water, soil, and potentially, in wildlife and people. Many
persistent toxics have been identified among these byproducts, including several of the "dirty dozen" POPs: dioxins
and furans, PCBs, and HCB. In 1994, the British manufacturer ICI Chemical and Polymers Limited concluded in an
internal memo that it was nearly impossible to avoid creating dioxins and furans during the manufacture of EDC.[90]

Some of these "dirty dozen" compounds may occur at
substantial levels. In 1995, for example, Greenpeace scientists examined the wastes from a Vulcan Materials EDC facility in the U.S. state of Louisiana, and concluded that the
plant's discharges were "among the most dioxin-contami-
nated wastes ever discovered." At a Dow Chemical plant also
in Louisiana, industry chemists found that PCBs accounted
for 0.03 percent of the plant's EDC heavy end wastes. That
may not sound like much, but if it's a typical level of contamination, then the world's PVC manufacturers may be producing several tons of PCBs unintentionally per year.[91]

The second step in the PVC recipe calls for heating the
EDC in the absence of oxygen. This process converts the EDC

to vinyl chloride monomer, or VCM. Like its precursor, VCM isn't a POP but it is dangerous. It's a carcinogen and a nerve poison. It has also been linked to liver damage, suppression of the immune system, and testicular abnormalities. VCM production also generates a substantial quantity of byproducts— by weight, byproducts account for about 3 percent of the results of VCM synthesis. Given current global rates of VCM production, several hundred thousand tons of these byproducts are generated every year. Nobody knows what exactly is in these materials, but they are likely to be contaminated by dioxins and furans. In 1998, scientists studying VCM byproducts at a fairly up-to-date Russian facility found them heavily contaminated with dioxins and furans.[92]

In the final stage of PVC synthesis, the VCM is liquified under pressure and then mixed with a chemical solution that causes the VCM molecules to link together into long chains, or polymers. The result is PVC, in the form of a fine, white powder. The process creates substantial waste, because of the spent mixture, but—as far as is known—no POPs are emitted at this stage.[93]

Unfortunately, raw PVC is practically useless, because the chlorine makes it brittle and prone to degrade rapidly when exposed to ultraviolet light. With other polymers, such problems can be dealt with by modifying their carbon chains, but with PVC, that approach doesn't work. Instead, various other chemicals must be added to the resin to give it the necessary durability and flexibility. These additives are not chemically bonded to the resin, so they may migrate to the surface of the material and leak into the surrounding environment. (Think of the smell of a new shower curtain: your nose is detecting the "out-gassing" of plastic additives.) As additives migrate out, PVC becomes brittle again, limiting its usefulness.[94]

Several different types of PVC additives are a health concern; heavy metals, for example, are sometimes used as stabilizers. But in terms of the quantities used, the most important additives are plasticizers, compounds that confer flexibility. Some 90 percent of plasticizers belong to a group of 25 compounds called phthalates, and some of the most common phthalates are POPs or POP-like compounds.[95]

Very roughly, global phthalate production appears to be in the range of 5.5 million tons a year. Because of their role in PVC production, phthalates are ubiquitous in both manufactured products and the environment. "It has become very difficult to analyze any soil or water sample without detecting phthalate esters," writes U.S. EPA scientist Robert Menzer, in a toxicology textbook. Phthalates have even been found in a species of deep sea jellyfish that lives 1,000 meters below the surface of the North Atlantic. Some experts argue that even supposedly pure laboratory materials may be contaminated with phthalates, making it difficult to establish baseline levels of exposure.[96]

In both wildlife and laboratory animals, phthalates have been linked to a range of reproductive health effects, including reduced fertility, miscarriage, birth defects, abnormal sperm counts, and testicular damage, as well as to liver and kidney cancer. As early as the 1970s, scientists had found that chicken embryos died when subjected to a 0.4 percent solution of one of the most common phthalates, diethylhexylphthalate (DEHP). That's a very high concentration by the standards of modern toxicology, but human blood stored in vinyl bags can reach this level in a day or two.[97]

Far more troubling are the low-dose effects of several phthalates. For example, EPA testing on laboratory animals has shown that *in utero* exposure to DEHP can deform the male sex organs and cause other types of "demasculinization," at levels far below those of previous toxicological concern. The same is true of another common phthalate, dibutyl phthalate.[98]

In humans, no "safe" level of exposure to phthalates has been determined, but numerous studies show that people are probably being contaminated by substantial quantities of these substances. For example, hospital patients receiving intravenous infusions have been shown to be at risk of exposure to DEHP, which can leach directly out of intravenous tubes and into the patients' bloodstreams. Recently, scientists at the U.S. Centers for Disease Control and Prevention have detected phthalates in urine from women of child-bearing age, at levels that cause fetal abnormalities in laboratory animals. And various studies have shown that children who chew on PVC toys—such as pacifiers and teething rings—absorb phthalates into their bodies.[99]

There is also growing evidence of actual injury. Swedish researchers recently reported that male workers in PVC plants have a risk of developing seminoma (a form of testicular cancer) that is six times that of the general population. The increased risk appears to be linked to DEHP, which can promote tumors by disrupting the endocrine system. (No increase in risk was found among workers manufacturing other types of plastics.) Another recent study found DEHP present at seven times the normal level in a group of Puerto Rican girls, aged 6 months to 2 years, who were showing premature breast development. A 1999 study in Oslo, Norway concluded that young children may absorb phthalates from vinyl floor covering; children in homes with such coverings had an 89 percent greater chance of developing bronchial obstruction and symptoms of asthma than did children living in homes with PVC-free floor coverings.[100]

Phthalates can leach out of intravenous tubes and into patients' bloodstreams.

At the end of its useful life, PVC is once again a source of POPs. PVC waste is already substantial and it's expected to grow considerably in the coming years. In the European Union alone, PVC waste is expected to jump 76 percent over the next two decades, from 4.1 million tons in 1999 to 7.2 million tons by 2020. There are at present three standard disposal options: incineration, dumping the material in landfills (the usual procedure for construction wastes), and more recently, recycling. None of these is a satisfactory long-term solution.[101]

Recycling might seem like the best approach, but recycling PVC is problematic due to its high additive and chlorine content. At recycling centers, incoming plastics are sorted, then crushed and pulverized. When a load with some PVC in it is treated this way, the various PVC formulations lose their chemical distinctiveness and contaminate any other plastics in the batch. The resulting bits of plastic may be uniform in size, but they are extremely varied in terms of additive content. (Another reprocessing strategy is to heat the materials, which breaks them down chemically into plastic monomers, oil-like compounds, and hydrochloric acid.)[102]

In essence, reprocessed PVC is downgraded. Such material can be used for products with very low performance standards, such as railroad ties, highway sound barriers, marine bulkheads, and construction "lumber" inside walls that are not load-bearing. It is estimated that two-thirds of current PVC demand could in theory be met with recycled PVC. But according to the Association of Postconsumer Plastic Recyclers (a U.S. plastic trade association), there are few markets for downgraded PVC. Even if there were viable markets, there is still the contamination factor. As one APPR board member put it, "the whole plastics recycling industry would run more smoothly if PVC was not part of the post-consumer waste packaging stream."[103]

Given the relatively low costs of landfilling and of virgin PVC, the current economics do not favor recycling. Recycling any plastic requires costly, labor-intensive sorting of enormous amounts of material. In New York City, for example, scores of workers manually separate plastic items from a *daily* stream of 2,000 tons of metals, glass, plastic, paper, and other materials. By volume, about 60 percent of post-consumer waste is mixed plastics but very little of that is PVC. The containers that consumers toss into their recycling bins are primarily high density polyethylene and polyethylene terephthalate. (In 1998, these materials accounted for 94 percent of all plastic bottles collected in the United States.) In the United States and Canada, just 0.1 percent of post-consumer PVC is now recycled. In the European Union, the figure stands at 3 percent. Since the early 1990s, waste PVC is increasingly being shipped to

China, India, or Africa for "reprocessing," where it is usually either just burned or buried.[104]

Worldwide, most PVC wastes are sent to landfills. In most European countries, for example, this share is between 50 and 90 percent. (Only Denmark reports less than 30 percent.) Yet PVC is only a tiny fraction of the total volume of municipal solid waste. In Europe, just 2.5 percent of total landfilled municipal waste is PVC. In Japan, the share is 12.2 percent. The share of chlorine that PVC contributes, however, is quite high: it accounts for up to 66 percent of chlorine in the household solid waste stream.[105]

Unregulated dumps are still common in much of the world, a condition that allows phthalates and other PVC additives to contaminate groundwater and air. Even in Europe, it wasn't until 1994 that leachate control systems were required for landfills. Open air dumps are most susceptible to leaching: about one-third of the phthalates will leak into the environment under aerobic conditions. And if the PVC is buried, it typically outlasts any collection system intended to prevent leaching. Even where state-of-the-art bottom liners and drainage pipes exist, the system is usually only guaranteed for about 80 years. Since rigid PVC does not have a half-life of any "relevant rate," in the words of an EU-commissioned study, its presence in the environment will continue long after the official life of a dump.[106]

As far as POPs are concerned, incineration is the worst waste disposal strategy of all. Yet a large portion of PVC-laden waste is simply burned. Given the material's chlorine content, that is a virtual guarantee of significant dioxin emissions. Worldwide, incineration of medical and municipal wastes, both of which usually include a substantial burden of PVC accounts for 69 percent of known dioxin and furan releases into the atmosphere—some 7,000 kilograms a year. (This figure is only a partial estimate, since it includes emissions for only the 15 countries that responded to a 1999 UNEP survey on the subject.)[107]

Japan currently reports the highest level of dioxin emissions in the world. The Japanese government is now trying

to contain dioxin releases from more than 3,800 highly polluting municipal incinerators. (In contrast, the United States
has fewer than 200 such facilities in operation.) But Japan is
not the only country facing a dioxin crisis from incineration:
on a per capita basis, the emissions rate for the Netherlands
is almost as high and the rate for Belgium is more than double. Many countries have only recently begun to monitor
emissions, and have yet to attempt to control them.
Reflecting on the public health implications of this practice,
a California nurse recently remarked, "I came to the chilling
realization that the trash I throw away on my unit is actually causing people to get the cancer and reproductive problems which I'm then treating."[108]

New evidence suggests that an enormous quantity of
dioxin is being produced by the unregulated burning of
household waste in open pits or in barrels in the backyard.
The high emissions result from a large proportion of PVC in
the waste and low burning temperatures. The first dioxin
assessment conducted by the Commission for Environmental Cooperation of the North American Free Trade
Agreement found that half of Mexico's emissions may come
from the burning of household waste. In the United States, a
recent study showed that three dozen households that
burned their trash outdoors emitted as much in the way of
dioxins and furans as a "properly operated waste incinerator
serving up to 120,000 households." These findings have
troubling implications for rural areas, especially in developing countries, where a great deal of waste is burned in the
open. Such concerns led the Philippines to ban all waste
incineration in 1999.[109]

There is, however, a point of controversy here. Some
researchers have pointed out that there is no clear relationship between the dioxin and furan emissions coming out of
an incinerator and the chlorine content of the waste going
into it. This is because many other factors influence the production of dioxins: the temperature of the burn, the oxygen
level, the availability of surfaces on which dioxin formation
can occur, and so on. It is also true that many apparently

innocuous substances may sometimes produce dioxins when burned—wood, for instance, or table salt. But while there is a continuum of sorts, there are nevertheless huge differences of degree. According to tests conducted by the German EPA in 1991, PVC combustion produces dioxins in ash in the range of 7.5 to 662 ppt (parts per trillion), while the results for paper, wood, or cotton containing inorganic chloride were below the detection limit of 0.1 ppt. Removing PVC from the incinerator waste stream won't end dioxin production, but it will certainly result in a substantial reduction.[110]

Soybean oil makes a better plasticizer than phthalates.

Faced with such risks, a growing number of policy makers and consumers are looking to change the role of PVC in their lives. What they are finding is that alternatives are currently available for almost every application of PVC. In 1997, for example, a consulting firm hired by the Canadian government produced a cost-benefit analysis for 90 percent of Canada's PVC uses, including pipes, siding, window frames, wire and cables, flooring, and various applications in flexible materials. (See Table 4.) Since construction accounts for 60 percent of PVC use, building codes may provide an especially important point of leverage: as it becomes economically feasible to do so, requiring materials other than PVC for new projects could give substitution efforts an enormous boost.[111]

The substitute materials themselves vary widely. Some are a direct throwback to an earlier era, such as wooden window frames. Others are high-tech modifications of familiar materials, such as the new biopolymers that are being produced from common crops. In general, the challenge will be to move away from the current, minimize-the-up-front-cost response to our material needs, and to adopt a more sophisticated approach, which seeks to minimize the *total* cost, both economic and environmental.

One potentially useful strategy is to alter the composition of PVC itself. For example, there is a group of compounds derived from various vegetable oils that can be used

TABLE 4

Alternatives to Major Construction Uses of PVC, According to a 1997 Canadian Study

Application	Alternatives (primary first) (secondary in italics)	Change in Cost if Alternatives Were Used	Change in Cost of the Application's Total Sales
		(1997 Canadian dollars)[1]	(percent)
Pipes	HDPE or ABS plastic	+44 million	+2
	Ductile iron, concrete, or copper/cast iron	*+96 million*	*+5*
Siding	Aluminum	+80 million	+10
Window frames	Wood	-118 million	-10
	Aluminum	*+55 million*	*+5.3*
Cable insulation	Polyethylene plastic	+181 million	+11
Flooring	Polyolefin plastic	+338 million	+11
	Ceramic tile and alternative carpeting	*+426 million*	*+14*

[1]Canadian dollars were not converted to U.S. dollars because of substantial exchange rate variation ($1 Cdn was $0.74 U.S. in January 1997 but $0.66 in October 2000).
Source: See endnote 111.

to plasticize PVC. In effect, soybean oil can substitute for phthalates. In the United States, vegetable oil plasticizers represented about 15 percent of the market for phthalates in 1996. Although they are generally more expensive than phthalates, they have several properties that phthalates lack: they confer stability, thereby eliminating the need for heavy metal stabilizers, and they do not leach out of the plastic, so they extend the life of the product.[112]

There may be other ways to make PVC safer. A

Canadian company, for example, has recently designed a PVC filler from calcium hydroxide. This material is intended to prevent phthalates from leaching and to neutralize the hydrochloric acid that forms when PVC is burned. Should the filler itself prove safe, adding it to the PVC recipe could be a useful stop-gap measure, until the time that non-PVC substitutes are in place.[113]

Of course, the more effective strategy over the long-term will be to identify whole-material substitutes for PVC. It's interesting to note that as early as 1971, NASA scientists were warning against the use of PVC in aerospace because of its volatility in a vacuum and the presence of phthalates. Moreover, as a NASA engineer noted in a letter to the editors of *Chemical and Engineering News,* "substitute polymers... are available and in many cases they have far superior physical properties at a small sacrifice in immediate cost."[114]

In general, the simplest solution may be simply to turn to another conventional plastic. Fortunately, not all plastics are as bad as PVC. The most common plastic in the world, polyethylene, just happens to be the one that the international environmental group Greenpeace considers to be the least harmful of the petroleum-based plastics. Because of their simpler polymer structures, polyethylene and the closely related polypropylene require no plasticizers and need fewer additives than PVC. (Polyethylene is also much cheaper than PVC—about one-tenth the environmental cost per unit weight.)[115]

Replacing PVC with nonchlorinated plastics such as polyethylene virtually eliminates the chances of forming POPs. A new generation of polyolefins (the class of plastics to which polyethylene and polypropylene belong) is being developed that may be custom tailored to meet many of the current applications of PVC, often using the same processing equipment.[116]

Perhaps even more visionary is the interest in producing plastic resins from plants. This is actually how the original plastics were made; for example, sap from the Malaysian *Gutta percha* tree was used to make the plastic that insulated telegraph wires in the 19th century. Today such biopolymers are derived from a wide variety of plant materials—oat hulls, corn, soybeans, oil seeds, or wood. In the United States, some federal funding is now available for research on biopolymers and some large corporations are showing interest in the possibilities. In April 2000, for example, Cargill Dow announced plans to build a large factory for turning out plastic from corn. The potential of this line of development could be substantial: the crops could be grown organically and processed in a closed-loop manufacturing system with renewable energy sources, yielding a virtually nonpolluting plastic.[117]

At present, unfortunately, the possibilities for substituting biopolymers for PVC are fairly limited. Because of their fragility, the current starch-based resins are generally only suitable for short-lived items, and most PVC is used for durable applications. But as with other environmental technologies, there is reason to hope that demand will help drive innovation. Growing concerns about PVC are likely to mean substantial profits for any company that succeeds in developing biopolymers to replace it. And in the meantime, there are some important short-term opportunities—for example, replacing PVC in medical goods. Such applications have important implications for public health; the sooner PVC is phased out of products like intravenous tubing, the better.[118]

The relationship between PVC and dangerous chemicals is complicated: POPs and POP-like materials are byproducts throughout the PVC lifecycle, from manufacture, to use, to disposal. The politics of PVC is complicated as well. Any serious effort to phase it out will likely encounter opposition not just from the industry that produces it, but from at least some segments of the industries that use it in large quantities.

But there is a useful strategic lesson hidden within all this complexity: complicated processes are susceptible to change at many different points. It should be possible to develop an agenda that pursues an array of substitution strategies simultaneously, while looking for business and political opportunities to help speed the transition. Perhaps some of those strategies will turn out to be dead ends. But by developing a "complex solution" to fit a complex problem, it should be possible to reach the goal—the replacement of PVC—even though the exact means of achieving it are likely to be in flux.

Leveraging Change

The POPs treaty negotiations could mark a significant turning point in humanity's relationship with synthetic chemicals. Politicians, business leaders, activists, and concerned citizens can use the treaty process as an opportunity to build support for the precautionary principle. We can move from a posture of acceptance and end-of-pipe control, to one that questions the need for toxics in the first place and that seeks safer alternatives. The groundwork for such a transition is already being built. Countries are implementing trade bans, emissions registries, and taxes on toxic materials. Some companies are redesigning production processes. Consumers are insisting on safer products. These activities alone will not achieve a phaseout of POPs and other dangerous industrial chemicals, but they will help spur broad development of cost effective and viable nontoxic substitutes. A fundamental change in the chemical economy is within reach.[119]

The key to using the treaty process effectively is to accept the goal endorsed by Klaus Töpfer and many other officials involved in the POPs treaty process. When the UNEP Executive Director called for "the elimination of POPs, not simply their better management," he set a standard by which the treaty itself will ultimately be judged. Adopting a hard line on this issue is one of the primary challenges that treaty delegates face.[120]

Currently, 15 countries of the more than 120 involved in the talks are adamantly opposed to the language of eventual elimination, particularly with respect to unintentional byproducts. This minority camp includes several major chemical producers: the United States, Japan, and South Korea. These nations argue that reducing POPs is a sufficient response to the problem. But most European nations, India, and a majority of other countries have come out in favor of eventual elimination.[121]

A compromise on this central point could render the treaty practically meaningless. Moreover, such a position could jeopardize standards already incorporated into existing regional agreements, which essentially laid the treaty's foundation. For instance, the 1998 OSPAR Strategy on Hazardous Substances commits its Northeast Atlantic signatories to stopping emissions of hazardous substances by 2020, a so-called "generational goal." Although its primary purpose is to protect the marine environment, the agreement has far-reaching implications for land-based activities as well. And it's obviously relevant to any broad attempt to regulate POPs.[122]

Further complicating the treaty process is the challenge of paying for the phaseout and safe disposal of POPs, and for the development of alternatives. An assistance fund has been established but to date, only a few industrial countries have pledged money for it. The treaty's financial mechanism has yet to take shape, but it will be crucial to incorporate a financial safety net for communities struggling to rid themselves of POPs. And the financial issue is connected to the elimination issue: over the long term, complete elimination of POPs is far more cost-effective than reduction, since elimination also does away with expenditures associated with hazardous waste.[123]

In response to the nearly universal recognition of the need to expand the treaty beyond the original "dirty dozen" substances, a group of experts has been working on the criteria for adding other POPs once the treaty comes into effect (in 2003 at the earliest). The group has benefited from a recently completed regional agreement on POPs, the Aarhus Protocol to the 1979 Convention on Long-Range Transboundary Air Pollution, which was signed by 55 members of the U.N. Economic Commission of Europe. (See Table 5.) The protocol sets limits for half-life in air (a surrogate measure of the potential for long-range transport), bioaccumulation, persistence, and toxicity. Establishing such standards in the treaty is critical to ensuring that it become a living document with a long useful life, and not simply an attempt to regulate a small group of chemicals, most of which are already heavily restricted. (See Table 6.)[124]

But there should be some flexibility in deciding what other substances to include. For example, the persistence of a substance is not a set value but a trait that varies in response to environmental conditions. An approach consistent with the precautionary principle would take such variation into account. Exhaustive proof of a substance's eligibility for listing should not be required. Instead, the treaty should state that the lack of scientific certainty will not, in itself, be grounds to exclude a chemical. Even if a substance falls short by one measure, it may still merit inclusion if it scores high by other criteria.[125]

An analysis by the U.S. EPA identified some likely candidates for future attention, based on the toxicity of their breakdown products and their tendency to bioaccumulate: the insecticides chlordecone and isodrin, the fungicide methyl mercury, octachlorostyrene (a chemical used in reinforced plastics and rubber manufacturing), and polybrominated biphenyls or PBBs (flame retardants in plastics and electronics). The Aarhus Protocol lists PAHs in general, the insecticides chlordecone and lindane, hexabromobiphenyl (a type of PBB), and three heavy metals with the 12 UNEP POPs. Clearly, there are numerous compounds besides the "dirty dozen" that deserve scrutiny.[126]

Regardless of how negotiators resolve these issues, there are numerous opportunities to phase out questionable substances right now, without waiting for the treaty to be ratified. Anna Lindh, then Sweden's Minister for the Environment, observed in 1995: "The question is not whether to phase out PVC, but how to phase it out." World leaders have begun to ask the same question about many other dangerous substances.[127]

TABLE 5

Selected International Conventions Complementary to the POPs Treaty

Aarhus Protocol on Persistent Organic Pollutants to the Long-Range Transboundary Air Pollution Convention, June 1998

Strengths:	• Covers 16 POPs; bans 8, restricts 4, and calls for phaseout of others
	• Includes specific criteria for adding chemicals
	• Includes Western and Eastern Europe, Canada, Russia, and the United States
Weaknesses:	• No developing countries involved
	• Covers air pollution only, not soil or water pollution
Status:	• 5 parties; 11 more needed

Rotterdam Convention on the Prior Informed Consent (PIC) Procedure for Certain Hazardous Chemicals and Pesticides in International Trade, September 1998

Strengths:	• Creates an information exchange procedure on national bans and restrictions to reduce imports of unwanted, harmful chemicals
	• Covers 7 POPs among a total of 5 industrial chemicals and 22 pesticides
Weaknesses:	• No enforcement "teeth" until ratified—voluntary procedure until then
	• No global record of shipments
Status:	• 11 parties; 39 more needed

Basel Convention on the Control of Transboundary Movements of Hazardous Wastes and their Disposal, 1989, and 1995 Amendment

Strengths:	• Most POPs qualify as hazardous wastes when destined for final deposition or recycling
	• Singles out wastes contaminated with PCBs, dioxins, and furans
	• Technical cooperation trust fund established to assist developing countries in implementation
	• 1995 amendment will stop exports of hazardous waste from OECD countries to non-OECD countries
	• Legally binding with criminal penalties
Weaknesses:	• Applies to imports only, not production or use
	• Amendment not in force yet
Status:	• Convention: entered into force May 1992; 141 parties
	• 1995 Amendment: 21 parties; 41 more needed

Source: See endnote 124.

In June 1999, for example, President Joseph Estrada of the Philippines set a historic precedent by signing the world's first national ban on all waste incineration. The law received strong support from environmentalists, community activists, and the Philippines Department of Environment and Natural Resources, which had called for such a ban. The agency argued that composting and recycling should be the standard waste handling procedures, and that nonburning technologies like microwaving should be used to sterilize medical wastes and other biohazardous materials. In a similar move, incineration was recently banned in Costa Rica by President Miguel Echeverría. Notwithstanding the difficulties in implementing such far-reaching policies, high-profile decisions like these set an important tone for consumers, manufacturers, and regulators: they reinforce the notion that change can happen quickly and that public health and environmental concerns can transcend economic interest, narrowly defined.[128]

The current debate in Europe concerning phthalates illustrates the importance of such thinking. Although public concern over phthalates dates back nearly 15 years in northern Europe, it was not until July 2000 that the European Parliament voted to permanently ban all phthalate softeners from PVC toys and other items that children are likely to chew on. Pending approval by the Council of Ministers, "this vote should pave the way for an EU-wide ban which has so far been opposed by a few Member States," according to Greenpeace International. (Eight European nations have unilaterally banned the additives in PVC toys for toddlers.) Although limited to just one of PVC's many applications, an EU ban would loom large in the global market, challenging manufacturers on the Continent and abroad to make safer toys or lose market share.[129]

Dealing with such trade issues will be critical to getting a handle on POPs. There is an important precedent for this effort, in the form of bans on hazardous waste imports. By 1997, more than 100 countries had enacted such bans, which now cover much of the developing world, including all of

TABLE 6

Regulatory Status of the "Dirty Dozen" POPs

Chemical	Countries with Bans[1]	Countries with Restrictions[2]	Countries with Import Bans
Aldrin	72	10	52
Chlordane	57	17	33
DDT	60	26	46
Dieldrin	67	9	53
Endrin	65	9	7
Heptachlor	59	17	36
Hexachlorobenzene	59	9	4
Mirex	52	10	0
Toxaphen	58	12	0
PCBs	9	4	5
Dioxins	0	23	0
Furans	0	22	0

[1]Bans are a complete prohibition of a use; they may cover all uses or just the principal use. Both national laws and EC regulations are included.   [2]Restrictions are national laws that impose conditions on a use but that do not ban it outright.
Source: See endnote 124.

Africa, the South Pacific, and Central America. Much of Asia, however, remains wide open. Certainly, hazardous waste includes many materials that are not POPs, but several recent international agreements on the waste trade explicitly include these compounds and that helps set the stage for further action. (See Table 5.) Although they are not yet in force, the Prior Informed Consent (PIC) procedure of the Rotterdam Convention and the similar 1995 Amendment to the Basel Convention have considerable potential in this regard.[130]

The crux of the PIC procedure is its requirement that exporting countries share with prospective importing countries any available scientific, technical, or economic information about the chemicals being shipped, including an account of any bans or restrictions within the country of origin concerning such materials. The destination countries have the authority to decide whether or not to accept the shipments and the senders are obligated to comply with these decisions. The 1995 amendment to the Basel Convention takes this power of refusal to another level. Once it comes into force, it will prohibit any shipments of hazardous waste from OECD countries to non-OECD countries. A blanket ban such as this will not only make it easier to detect illegal shipments, but will in theory force industrialized nations (typically the generators of hazardous waste) to deal with their own waste problems—a useful incentive to industrial reform.[131]

These two procedures are a huge step in the direction of precautionary chemicals management. The next logical step is to take this approach beyond trading procedures, to the public at large. Accurate information about the production, toxicology, and regulatory status of dangerous chemicals should be freely available to everyone. The idea that people should have the right to know what they are being exposed to dates back at least 16 years. In the wake of the 1984 Bhopal, India disaster, environmentalists, community activists, and the U.S. EPA successfully lobbied the U.S. Congress to pass the world's first community right-to-know law, over strong protests from industry officials. The 1986 Emergency Planning and Community Right-to-Know Act created a national database of toxic emissions from factories. Known as the Toxic Release Inventory (TRI), its data allow citizens, companies, and the media to publicize the worst polluters and to bring public attention to toxic waste issues. The TRI does not cover all toxic chemicals or all sources of pollution (many POPs are not included on the current list of 600 reportable chemicals). But it has proven extremely useful and the idea is catching on elsewhere.[132]

Today, seven industrial countries and one developing nation—Mexico—have implemented systems similar to the TRI. Internationally known as Pollutant Release and Transfer Registers (PRTRs), they usually contain data on chemicals in

most facilities and in air, water, and soil. Several other countries—including Argentina, the Czech Republic, Egypt,
Japan, and five former Soviet Union nations—are expected
to adopt similar systems soon. In addition to tracking emissions, these registers are an important tool for developing
national POPs inventories, as called for in the draft POPs
treaty. In combination with the PIC procedures, they help
reduce corporate secrecy, encourage greater public participa-
tion, and provide a check against government and corporate
abuses.[133]

At least one jurisdiction has found that simply demand-
ing this type of information can change corporate behavior.
In 1989, the U.S. state of Massachusetts passed a Toxics Use
Reduction Act that requires major chemical users in the state
to produce a detailed toxics use reduction plan. The plan
must analyze the costs and benefits of both the toxics and the
alternatives; it must also show that a company understands
how it is using particular toxic chemicals, for what purpose,
and at what cost. (Some 1,420 industrial chemicals are listed
under the law.) There is no legal obligation to implement any
pollution prevention measures, only to study chemical use in
detail on a bi-yearly basis.[134]

But of the nearly 1,000 companies that have filed plans
to date, some 80 percent followed their own advice and
implemented alternatives. As a result, they have achieved
significant reductions in the amount of chemicals used to
manufacture a given quantity of product. And these reductions have not injured business: on average, production has
increased by one-third. (See Figure 7.) The companies have
also saved a total of $15 million in operating costs, exclusive
of the considerable human health and environmental benefits of such reductions.[135]

All these activities have set the stage for greater citizen
involvement. Consider, for example, the vibrant and vocal
NGO network that sprang up during the treaty negotiations.
Greenpeace scientist Pat Costner has noted that the more
than 200 NGOs represented in the International POPs
Elimination Network outnumber official delegates to the

FIGURE 7

Changes in Toxic Chemical Use Per Product Unit, Reported Under the Massachusetts Toxics Use Reduction Act, 1990–97

Percentage change per product unit

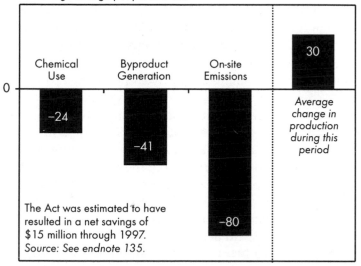

The Act was estimated to have resulted in a net savings of $15 million through 1997.
Source: See endnote 135.

treaty almost two to one. In some ways, this reflects the fact that the POPs issue has united two often disparate communities—environmentalists and biologists on the one hand, doctors and public health specialists on the other.[136]

Coalitions of this sort are not just changing diplomacy; in some cases, they can be more effective than governments in changing corporate practices. In the mid-1990s, for instance, Filipino citizens forced a French company to abandon its plans to build the world's largest waste incinerator just north of Manila. Elsewhere, in response to extensive lobbying by environmentalists and growing public concern, many companies, including General Motors, IKEA, Lego, and Nike, are pledging to go PVC-free. In the health care field, activists have collaborated with stockholders of medical equipment manufacturers to file shareholder resolutions expressing concern about the health risks of dioxin emissions from the incineration of PVC medical waste. Such actions have prompted several manufacturers to announce plans to stop using PVC in intravenous tubing, blood bags, and gloves. To meet growing demand, at least a dozen manufacturers in the United States now offer non-PVC medical supplies and equipment.[137]

Some corporations are apparently reacting to the shifting politics by adopting a "precautionary activism" of their own. In May 2000, for instance, the 3M Company announced that it would voluntarily stop making most of its Scotchgard stain-repellent products by year's end. One of Scotchgard's main ingredients comes from a group of chemicals called perfluorooctane sulfonates (PFOs), and while PFOs are not POPs, at least some of them are POP-like: they are highly persistent and pervasive in the environment. PFOs are used to repel water and oil on furniture and automobile upholstery, carpets, even food packaging. 3M agreed to the phaseout after discussing proprietary scientific findings with the U.S. EPA. Scotchgard accounts for about $320 million or 2 percent of the company's annual sales. Environmentalists and Clinton administration officials praised the company's decision to drop the chemicals even though risks to human health had not been proven.[138]

Such actions are encouraging, but the current track record of voluntary corporate agreements is mixed at best. In 1991, for example, the Danish EPA and the PVC industry agreed that the industry would voluntarily recycle 41 percent of PVC waste from the construction sector by 1995. (Used construction PVC is much easier to recycle than postconsumer PVC because it's relatively easy to sort and it contains little in the way of plasticizers.) But a follow-up analysis by the government in 1997 found that the industry had recycled just 10 to 15 percent of PVC waste, and much of that material was "downcycled" to low-grade uses, so there was no detectable net reduction in the consumption of virgin PVC. Many producers, such as those represented by the International Council of Chemical Associations, argue that

POPs can be managed without regulations or bans. The Danish experience suggests that corporate voluntarism is important but not in itself an adequate strategy for moving beyond POPs.[139]

Changes in production methods are critical, but it's not reasonable to put the full burden of this issue on manufacturing. The other side of the equation is reducing the demand for such products in the first place, especially in industrial countries. Each year, for example, the United States sends more paper to landfills than China consumes. Even in the developing countries, per capita consumption of PVC, pesticides, and paper is expected to jump dramatically in the coming years. Consumer responsibility is as important as manufacturer responsibility.[140]

One way to encourage a shift from dangerous chemicals to safer practices is to tax the offending substance or merely reduce tax exemptions for it. A noteworthy precedent in this connection is Denmark's recently imposed tax on PVC and phthalates. Similar efforts have been undertaken with pesticides. Sweden, for instance, imposes a pesticide tax which consists of a 7.5 percent surcharge for every kilogram of active ingredient purchased. This levy was one of a set of government initiatives that helped Swedish farmers cut their pesticide use by 65 percent from 1986 to 1993. In Great Britain, some economists have suggested that a 30-percent tax on pesticides could result in use reductions on the order of 8 to 20 percent. The U.K. government is considering a pesticide tax whose rate would be determined by the level of hazard—the more toxic a pesticide is, the higher the tax on it would be. In the United States, a study by the environmental NGO Friends of the Earth found that of the $8.8 billion spent in 1997 on pesticides, nearly $276 million in government revenue was lost due to exemptions from state sales taxes. These public revenues could have helped fund research and development programs for IPM and organic farming.[141]

The complementary strategy is to offer tax breaks for alternative technologies, which are often expensive to imple-

ment even though their long-term environmental and economic benefits are clear. Tax breaks for TCF paper production, organic farming, and the use of non-PVC construction
materials could help scale up these approaches to a point
where they could become industry standards.[142]

Of course, individual consumer demand will have to
change as well. What does "overconsumption" mean to
most people? To judge from the ways in which the issue is
most commonly discussed, people who admit the legitimacy
of the issue are most likely to think in terms of visible degradation of the environment—of clearcut forests, overflowing
landfills, or enormous open-pit mines. But the invisible
degradation may just be as bad: we are living in a soup of
synthetic poisons and this too is in part the result of overconsumption.

We do not understand the risks that this form of overconsumption creates, but we do know that those risks are
grave and that they will burden many future generations.
That's why we need to find a place for the precautionary
principle within the realm of personal choice—within the
everyday decisions that in large measure make up our lives.
Reconciling personal consumption with social awareness is
perhaps one of the greatest challenges of our era. That effort
might begin with the kind of question used to advance the
precautionary principle within the chemical economy as a
whole. What do we really need? The answer will obviously
depend on individual tastes and circumstances. But as the
Massachusetts law has shown, there is much to be gained
simply by studying one's actions. Do we "need" to consume
POPs and similar chemicals? As our knowledge of the risks
and the alternatives continues to strengthen, it becomes
increasingly clear that the answer to that question is no.

Notes

1.   Michael A. Gallo and John Doull, "History and Scope of Toxicology," in Mary O. Amdur, John Doull, and Curtis D. Klaassen, eds., *Casarett and Doull's Toxicology: The Basic Science of Poisons*, 4th ed. (New York: Pergamon Press, 1991); Donald J. Ecobichon, "Toxic Effects of Pesticides," in ibid.; Ruth Norris, et al., *Pills, Pesticides, and Profits: The International Trade in Toxic Substances* (Croton-on-Hudson, NY: North River Press, 1982); Jeffrey L. Meikle, *American Plastic: A Cultural History* (New Brunswick, NJ: Rutgers University Press, 1997); and Christopher Flavin, *The Future of Synthetic Materials: The Petroleum Connection*, Worldwatch Paper No. 36 (Washington, DC: Worldwatch Institute, April 1980).

2.   Flavin, op. cit. note 1, and Joe Thornton, *Pandora's Poison: Chlorine, Health, and a New Environmental Strategy* (Cambridge, MA: MIT Press, 2000).

3.   Ted Schettler et al., *Generations at Risk: Reproductive Health and the Environment* (Cambridge, MA: MIT Press, 1999); Environmental Defense Fund (EDF), *Toxic Ignorance: The Continuing Absence of Basic Health Testing for Top-Selling Chemicals in the United States* (New York: EDF, 1997); Sanjoy Hazarika, *Bhopal: The Lessons of a Tragedy* (New Delhi: Penguin Books India, 1987); and Hilary French, *Vanishing Borders: Protecting the Planet in the Age of Globalization* (New York: W.W. Norton & Company, 2000). Recent studies: Jocelyn Kaiser, "Hazards of Particles, PCBs Focus of Philadelphia Meeting," *Science*, 21 April 2000; S. Patandin et al., "Effects of Environmental Exposure to Polychlorinated Biphenyls and Dioxins on Cognitive Abilities in Dutch Children at 42 Months of Age," *Journal of Pediatrics*, January 1999; Joseph L. Jacobson, and Sandra W. Jacobson, "Intellectual Impairment in Children Exposed to Polychlorinated Biphenyls *in Utero*," *New England Journal of Medicine*, 12 September 1996; Eric Dewailly et al., "Susceptibility to Infections and Immune Status in Inuit Infants Exposed to Organochlorines," *Environmental Health Perspectives*, March 2000. Pierre Ayotte, professor of toxicology, Department of Social Medicine and Prevention, Laval University, Quebec City, Québec, conversation with author, 27 October 2000.

4.   Donald MacKay, "Environmental Fate and Modeling of Long-Distance Atmospheric Transport of POPs," presentation at Harvard University School of Public Health, "Persistent Organic Pollutants (POPs): A Public Health Perspective," Cambridge, MA, 16–18 June 1999; Donald MacKay, Director, Environmental Modelling Center, Trent University, Peterborough, Ontario, Canada, e-mail to author, 24 September 1999; and EDF, op. cit. note 3. Three per day: U.S. EPA, *Toxic Substances Control Act at Twenty* (Washington, DC: fall 1996).

5.   The compound, 2,3,7,8-Tetrachlorodibenzo-*p*-Dioxin, or TCDD, is the prototype for a large family of dioxin and furan congeners that exhibit similar actions. In this paper, unless otherwise specified, the term "dioxins and furans" refers to TCDD mixtures. See Linda S. Birnbaum "TEFs: A Practical Approach to a Real-World Problem," *Human and Ecological Risk Assessment*, vol. 5, no. 1 (1999), and Robert Ayres, "The Life-Cycle of Chlorine, Part 1,"

Journal of Industrial Ecology, vol. 1, no. 1 (1997). For the treaty, see International Institute for Sustainable Development (IISD), "The Second Session of the International Negotiating Committee for an International Legally Binding Instrument for Implementing International Action on Certain Persistent Organic Pollutants (POPS): 25–29 January 1999, A Brief History of the POPs Negotiations," *Earth Negotiations Bulletin*, 1 February 1999; United Nations Environmental Programme (UNEP), "Report of the Intergovernmental Negotiating Committee for an International Legally Binding Instrument for Implementing International Action on Certain Persistent Organic Pollutants on the Work of Its Third Session, Geneva, 6–11 September 1999," (Geneva: 17 September 1999). Sources for Table 1: introduction dates from Terry Gips, *Breaking the Pesticide Habit: Alternatives to 12 Hazardous Pesticides* (Penang, Malaysia: International Alliance for Sustainable Agriculture and International Organization of Consumers Unions, 1990); and Paul Johnston, David Santillo, and Ruth Stringer, "Marine Environmental Protection, Sustainability and the Precautionary Principle," *Natural Resources Forum*, May 1999; dioxins and furans from UNEP, Chemicals Division, *Dioxin and Furan Inventories: National and Regional Emissions of PCDD/PCDF* (Geneva: Inter-Organization Programme for the Sound Management of Chemicals, May 1999); uses from Physicians for Social Responsibility, "International Effort Would Phase Out 12 Toxins," *PSR Monitor*, February 1998, and from L. Ritter et al., "An Assessment Report on: DDT-Aldrin-Dieldrin-Endrin-Chlordane-Heptachlor-Hexachlorobenzene-Mirex-Toxaphene, Polychlorinated Biphenyls, Dioxins and Furans prepared for the Inter-Organization Programme for the Sound Management of Chemicals" (Guelph, Ontario: Canadian Network of Toxicology Centres, December 1995).

6. Töpfer quote from UNEP, "Report of the Intergovernmental Negotiating Committee for an International Legally Binding Instrument for Implementing International Action on Certain Persistent Organic Pollutants on the Work of Its First Session, Montreal, 29 June–3 July 1998," (Geneva: 3 July 1998); UNEP, "Elimination of 10 Intentionally Produced Persistent Organic Pollutants Favoured by Treaty Negotiators: Health Need for DDT Exemption Seen," press release (Geneva: 13 September 1999); World Wide Fund for Nature (WWF), "Persistent Organic Pollutants Treaty: Eight Down, Four To Go," press release (Gland, Switzerland: 11 September 1999). Estimates from Michael Walls, Senior Counsel, Chemical Manufacturers Association, Arlington, VA, discussion with author, 17 September 1999, and from Pat Costner, Senior Scientist, Greenpeace International, e-mail to author, 20 September 1999.

7. "Government Ducks North Sea Deal on PCB Phase-Out," *ENDS Report*, February 1999; and Don Hinrichsen, *Coastal Waters of the World: Trends, Threats, and Strategies* (Washington, DC: Island Press: 1998).

8. Mobility from Frank Wania and Don MacKay, "Global Distillation," *Our Planet*, March 1997; from Wania and MacKay, "Global Fractionation and Cold Condensation of Low Volatility Organochlorine Compounds in Polar Regions," *Ambio*, February 1993. Distribution from Bommanna G.

Loganathan and Kurunthachalam Kannan, "Global Organochlorine Contamination Trends: An Overview," *Ambio*, May 1994; Staci L. Simonich and Ronald A. Hites, "Global Distribution of Persistent Organochlorine Compounds," *Science*, 29 September 1995 (tree bark); T. Colborn and M.J. Smolen, "Epidemiological Analysis of Persistent Organochlorine Contaminants in Cetaeceans," *Reviews of Environmental Contamination and Toxicology*, vol. 146 (1996); M.L. Lyke, "Toxin Threatens a Wonder of the Northwest," *Washington Post*, 8 November 1999; Bo Jansson et al., "Chlorinated and Brominated Persistent Organic Compounds in Biological Samples from the Environment," *Environmental Toxicology and Chemistry*, vol. 12 (1993); Thornton, op. cit. note 2. Ninety percent exposure from Arnold Schecter, "Exposure Assessment: Measurement of Dioxins and Related Chemicals in Human Tissues," in Arnold Schecter, ed., *Dioxins and Health* (New York: Plenum Press, 1994). For human contamination see Greenpeace International, *Unseen Poisons: Levels of Organochlorine Chemicals in Human Tissues* (Amsterdam: June 1998); Theo Colborn, "Restoring Children's Birthrights," *Our Planet*, March 1997; and Matthew P. Longnecker, Walter J. Rogan, and George Lucier, "The Human Health Effects of DDT (Dichlorodiphenyltrichloroethane) and PCBs (Polychlorinated Biphenyls) and an Overview of Organochlorines in Public Health," *Annual Review of Public Health*, vol. 18 (1997).

9.   Amdur, Doull, and Klaassen, op. cit. note 1; Rene P. Schwarzenbach, Philip M. Gschwend, and Dieter M. Imboden, *Environmental Organic Chemistry* (New York: John Wiley & Sons, 1993); and Thornton, op. cit. note 2.

10.   Amdur, Doull, and Klaassen, op. cit. note 1; U.S. National Research Council (NRC), *Hormonally Active Agents in the Environment* (Washington, DC: National Academy Press, prepublication copy, July 1999); Francoise Brucker-David, "Effects of Environmental Synthetic Chemicals on Thyroid Function," *Thyroid*, vol. 8, no. 9 (1998); U.S. EPA, *Dioxin: Scientific Highlights from Draft Reassessment (2000)*, Information Sheet 2 (Washington, DC: Office of Research and Development, 12 June 2000). Exposure limit for TCDD inferred from WHO, "WHO Experts Re-Evaluate Health Risks from Dioxins," press release WHO/45 (Geneva: 3 June 1998).

11.   Claes Bernes, Swedish Environmental Protection Agency, <sweionet. environ.se/issues/pop/pop.html>, viewed 5 October 2000; Amdur, Doull, and Klaassen, op. cit. note 1, and Thornton, op. cit. note 2.

12.   Robert C. Rhew, Benjamin R. Miller, and Ray F. Weiss, "Natural Methyl Bromide and Methyl Chloride Emissions from Coastal Salt Marshes," *Nature*, 20 January 2000. Chlorine in commerce from Robert Ayres, "The Life-Cycle of Chlorine, Part I: Chlorine Production and the Chlorine-Mercury Connection," *Journal of Industrial Ecology*, vol. 1, no. 1 (1997); and Ivan Amato, "The Crusade Against Chlorine," *Science*, 9 July 1993. Stearns quote from Amato, "The Crusade To Ban Chlorine," *Garbage*, summer 1994. Additional information on properties of chlorine from Lawrence J. Fisher, "Chlorinated Compounds: Research or Ban?"

Health & Environment Digest, May 1994.

13. Rebecca Renner, "What Fate for Brominated Fire Retardants?" *Environmental Science & Technology*, 1 May 2000; Jacob de Boer, et al., "Do Flame Retardants Threaten Ocean Life?" *Nature*, 2 July 1998; and Amdur, Doull, and Klaassen, op. cit. note 1.

14. WWF and the World Conservation Union (IUCN), *Creating a Sea Change* (Gland, Switzerland: October 1998).

15. Cheryl Siegel Scott and V. James Cogliano, "Trichloroethylene Health Risks: State of the Science," *Environmental Health Perspectives*, Supplement 2, May 2000; Daniel Wartenberg, Daniel Reyner, and Cheryl Siegel Scott, "Trichloroethylene and Cancer: Epidemiologic Evidence," *Environmental Health Perspectives*, Supplement 2, May 2000; and Chieh Wu and John Schaum, "Exposure Assessment of Trichloroethylene," *Environmental Health Perspectives*, Supplement 2, May 2000. Toxicity of breakdown products from Thornton, op. cit. note 2. OSPAR Convention for the Protection of the Marine Environment of the North-East Atlantic, "OSPAR Strategy with regard to Hazardous Substances," Ministerial Meeting of the OSPAR Commission (Sintra, Portugal: 22–23 July 1998); and J.J.M. Berdowski et al., "Technical Paper to the OSPAR-HELCOM-UNECE Emission Inventory of Heavy Metals and Persistent Organic Pollutants," (Delft, the Netherlands: TNO Institute of Environmental Sciences, 18 December 1995).

16. Schettler et al., op. cit. note 3; and Peter Eisler, "Government's Pesticide Review Lags," *USA Today*, 30 August 1999.

17. Jane Ellen Simmons, "Chemical Mixtures: Challenge for Toxicology and Risk Assessment," *Toxicology*, December 1995.

18. "Introduction: To Foresee and to Forestall," in Carolyn Raffensperger and Joel A. Tickner, eds., *Protecting Public Health and the Environment: Implementing the Precautionary Principle* (Washington, DC: Island Press, 1999); Carl F. Cranor, "Asymmetric Information, the Precautionary Principle, and Burdens of Proof," in ibid.; and Sheldon Krimsky, "The Precautionary Approach," *Forum for Applied Research and Public Policy*, fall 1998.

19. "Introduction," op. cit. note 18; Cranor, op. cit. note 18; and Krimsky, op. cit. note 18.

20. Janet N. Abramovitz and Ashley T. Mattoon, *Paper Cuts: Recovering the Paper Landscape*, Worldwatch Paper 149 (Washington, DC: Worldwatch Institute, December 1999).

21. Ibid; Figure 2 from ibid.

22. UNEP Chemicals Division, op. cit. note 5; Baltic and Great Lakes from Thornton, op. cit. note 2.

23. Abramovitz and Mattoon, op. cit. note 20.

24. World Bank Group, "Pulp and Paper Mills," in *Pollution Prevention and Abatement Handbook* (Washington, DC: July 1998), <wbln0018. worldbank.org/essd/essd.nsf/GlobalView/PPAH/$file/78-pulp.pdf>, viewed 22 September 2000; and "Roundtable on the Industrial Ecology of Pulp and Paper," *Journal of Industrial Ecology*, vol. 1, no. 3 (1998). Mechanical pulp capacity from International Institute for Environment and Development (IIED), *Towards a Sustainable Paper Cycle* (London: 1996).

25. FAO, *FAOSTAT Statistics Database*, <apps.fao.org>, viewed 5 October 2000. Chemical pulp capacity from IIED, op. cit. note 24.

26. Forty percent from FAO, op. cit. note 25.

27. Average pulp mill capacity from Thornton, op. cit. note 2; 35 tons from Abramovitz and Mattoon, op. cit. note 20; byproducts from Leena R. Suntio, Wan Ying Shiu, and Donald Mackay, "A Review of the Nature and Properties of Chemicals Present in Pulp Mill Effluents," *Chemosphere*, vol. 17, no. 7, 1988; and from Robert Ayres, "The Life Cycle of Chlorine, Part III: Accounting for Final Use," *Journal of Industrial Ecology*, vol. 2, no. 1 (1998); TRI data from U.S. EPA, "TRI Explorer: Industry Report, 1998" <www.epa.gov/cgibin/broker?view=UnitedStates&_program=xp_tri.sasmacr. tristart.macro>, viewed 9 August 2000; ranking in world from IIED, op. cit. note 24.

28. Ayres, op. cit. note 27; R. Lipkin, "Taking Chlorine Out of Tough Pollutants," *Science News*, 27 May 1995; Thornton, op. cit. note 2.

29. Peterson quote from Richard Stone, "Dioxins Dominate Denver Gathering of Toxicologists," *Science*, 18 November 1994. Janet Raloff, "Beyond Estrogens: Why Unmasking Hormone-Mimicking Pollutants Proves So Challenging," *Science News*, 15 July 1995. Florida from Stephen A. Bortone and William P. Davis, "Fish Intersexuality as Indicator of Environmental Stress," *Bioscience*, March 1994. Institute of Medicine, Committee of Evaluation of the Safety of Fishery Products, Food and Nutrition Board, *Seafood Safety* (Washington, DC: National Academy Press, 1991). U.S. EPA, Office of Water, "Update: National Listing of Fish and Wildlife Advisories" (Washington, DC: July 1999), <www.epa.gov/ost/fish/epafish.pdf>, viewed 6 October 2000.

30. Heron from Thomas Webster and Barry Commoner, "Overview: The Dioxin Debate," in Schecter, op. cit. note 8; gulls from Angel Lorenzen et al., "Relationships between Environmental Organochlorine Contaminant Residues, Plasma Corticosterone Concentrations, and Intermediary Metabolic Enzyme Activities in Great Lakes Herring Gull Embryos," *Environmental Health Perspectives*, March 1999, and Theo Colborn, Dianne Dumanoski, and John Peterson Myers, *Our Stolen Future* (New York: Penguin, 1996), and from Theo Colborn, Frederick S. vom Saal, and Ana M. Soto, "Developmental Effects of Endocrine-Disrupting Chemicals in Wildlife and

Humans," *Environmental Health Perspectives*, October 1993.

31. Carol Berger, "Canada's Once-Pristine North Tries to Curb Paper Mills' Waste," *Christian Science Monitor*, 17 October 1996; Sheila Polson, "Contaminated Fish Mean Loss of Culture to Penobscot Indians," *Christian Science Monitor*, 16 July 1996.

32. Mark P. Radka, "Policy and Institutional Aspects of the Sustainable Paper Cycle—An Asian Perspective," (Bangkok: UNEP, Regional Office for Asia and the Pacific, 1994). Ricardo Carrere and Larry Lohmann, *Pulping the South: Industrial Tree Plantations and the World Paper Economy* (Atlantic Highland, NJ: Zed Books Ltd., 1996).

33. IIED, op. cit. note 24, and FAO, op. cit. note 25. These are also the sources for Table 2.

34. Global production from Ashley T. Mattoon, "Paper Piles Up," in Lester R. Brown, Michael Renner, and Brian Halweil, *Vital Signs 2000* (New York: W.W. Norton & Company, 2000); Latin America from FAO, op. cit. note 25, and from Mark Payne, "Latin America Aims High for Next Century," *Pulp and Paper International*, August 1999. Asia from Hou-Main Chang, "Economic Outlook for Asia's Pulp and Paper Industry," *TAPPI Journal*, January 1999, available online at <www.tappi.org>; current Asian production from FAO, op. cit. note 25.

35. Carrere and Lohmann, op. cit. note 32; cost from Abramovitz and Mattoon, op. cit. note 20.

36. ECF from World Bank Group, op. cit. note 24; from "Cheaper Dioxin Controls Considered for Paper, Pulp," *Environmental Science & Technology*, 30 no. 9 (1996); and from "Roundtable on the Industrial Ecology of Pulp and Paper," op. cit. note 24. Equipment from Christoph Thies and Martin Kaiser, "It's Time to Clean Up Chlorine Bleaching," *Pulp and Paper International*, online edition, February 2000. Emissions comparison from Abramovitz and Mattoon, op. cit. note 20. Source for Figure 3: Alliance for Environmental Technology (AET), "Trends in World Bleached Chemical Pulp Production, 1990–1999," (January 2000) <www.aet.org/science/aet_trends_1999.html>, viewed 5 October 2000.

37. 1999 ECF statistics from AET, op. cit. note 36; U.S. pulp and paper production from FAO, op. cit. note 25. Chlorine consumption from Thornton, op. cit. note 2. Dioxin drop from Miller Freeman, Inc., *1999 North American Pulp and Paper Factbook* (San Francisco: 1998). U.S. EPA, "Fact Sheet: EPA's Final Pulp, Paper, and Paperboard 'Cluster Rule'—Overview," November 1997, EPA-821-F-97-010.

38. Thornton, op. cit. note 2. Effluent comparison from Abramovitz and Mattoon, op. cit. note 20; World Bank Group, op. cit. note 24.

39. World Bank Group, op. cit. note 24; Jay Ritchlin, "MillWatch Special Report: Reasons to Eliminate Chlorine Dioxide," (Vancouver: Reach for Unbleached! 30 June 1998), available online at <www.rfu.org>. "MNI-Malaysia's International Class Newsprint Mill Fully Operational in April 1999," *Malaysia Timber Bulletin*, vol. 4, no. 10, 1998. Scandinavia from Chlorine Free Products Association, *CFPA Today*, spring 1999. Six percent from AET, op. cit. note 36.

40. North America from Jurgen D. Kramer, "Pulping/Bleaching Technology View Shows North America Lagging," *Pulp and Paper*, 1 April 2000. European demand from Thies and Kaiser, op. cit. note 36.

41. Ken Geiser, "Cleaner Production and the Precautionary Principle," in Raffensperger and Tickner, op. cit. note 18.

42. United Parcel Service, "Reusable UPS Next Day Air Envelope Wins the Paperboard Packaging Council's Award," press release, 30 April 1998 available at <www.pressroom.ups.com/pressreleases/0,1014,235,00.html#235>, viewed 19 October 2000. Martin Koepenick, "L-P's Samoa Mill: An Environmental Performer," *Paper Age*, October 1998.

43. Grain production from Lester R. Brown, *Land, Man, and Food: Looking Ahead at World Food Needs*, Foreign Agriculture Economic Report No. 11 (Washington, DC: U.S. Department of Agriculture, November 1963); importance of major grains to human food supply from FAO, op. cit. note 25.

44. U.S. Department of Agriculture (USDA), *Production, Supply, and Distribution*, electronic database, (Washington, DC, updated September 2000); 2.5 million tons from David Pimentel, "Protecting Crops," in Wallace C. Olsen, ed., *The Literature of Crop Science* (Ithaca, NY: Cornell University Press, 1995).

45. Rachel Carson, *Silent Spring* (Boston: Houghton Mifflin, 1962); C.V. Bowen and S.A. Hall, "The Organic Insecticides," in USDA, *Insects: The Yearbook of Agriculture, 1952* (Washington, DC: USDA).

46. Carson, op. cit. note 45.

47. Production dates from Johnston et al., op. cit. note 5; Ritter et al., op. cit. note 5; and Gips, op. cit. note 5. HCB from Joint Canada-Philippines Planning Committee, "Annex II: Demonstration Substance Profiles," in *International Experts Meeting on Persistent Organic Pollutants: Towards Global Action*, meeting background report, Vancouver, Canada, 4–8 June 1995 (revised October 1995). Toxaphene from Susan T. Glassmeyer, David S. de Vault, and Ronald A. Hites, "Rates at Which Toxaphene Concentrations Decrease in Lake Trout from the Great Lakes," *Environmental Science & Technology*, vol. 34, no. 9 (2000). Fire ant from Nita A. Davidson and Nick D. Stone, "Imported Fire Ants," in Donald L. Dahlsten and Richard Garcia, eds., *Eradication of Exotic Pests: Analysis with Case Histories* (New Haven, CT: Yale University Press, 1989).

48. Country bans from UNEP, *Summary of Existing National Legislation on Persistent Organic Pollutants* (Geneva: 14 June 1999). DDT production and toxaphene from Intergovernmental Forum on Chemical Safety (IFCS), "Problems with Persistent Organic Pollutants: Towards Better Alternatives," IFCS Experts Meeting on POP, 17–19 June 1996, Manila, Philippines (Geneva: 6 June 1996), available at <irtpc.unep.ch.pops>; and Dev Raj, "India a Major Exporter of Killer Chemicals," *Environment Bulletin-India*, posted at <www.igc.org>, 17 November 1998. HCB from Joint Canada-Philippines Planning Committee, op. cit. note 47; and WWF Issue Brief, *Successful, Safe and Sustainable Alternatives to Persistent Organic Pollutants* (Gland, Switzerland: September 1999).

49. Global estimate based on cumulative production data cited in Johnston et al., op. cit. note 47; Alemayehu Wodageneh, "Trouble in Store," *Our Planet*, March 1997; FAO, "FAO Warns of the Dangerous Legacy of Obsolete Pesticides," press release (Rome: 24 May 1999).

50. Bark from Simonich and Hites, op. cit. note 8; breast milk from Longnecker, Rogan, and Lucier, op. cit. note 8.

51. Earlier pesticides from Montague Yudelman, Annu Ratta, and David Nygaard, *Pest Management and Food Production: Looking to the Future* (Washington, DC: IFPRI, September 1998); Congressional hearings from John H. Perkins, "Eradication: Scientific and Social Questions," in Dahlsten and Garcia, eds., op. cit., note 47, and from Schettler et al., op. cit. note 3.

52. Ecobichon, op. cit. note 1.

53. Ecobichon, op. cit. note 1. U.S. EPA, Office of Pesticide Programs, "Organophosphate Pesticides in Food: A Primer on Reassessment of Residue Limits," 735-F-99-014 (Washington, DC: EPA, May 1999) available online at <www.epa.gov/pesticides/op/primer.htm>, viewed 8 June 2000; and Schettler et al., op. cit. note 3.

54. "OPs and Parkinson's Disease," *Global Pesticide Campaign*, August 1999; and U.S. EPA, op. cit. note 53.

55. Edward Groth, Charles M. Benbrook, and Karen Lutz, "Update: Pesticides in Children's Foods, An Analysis of 1998 USDA PDP Data on Pesticide Residues," (Yonkers, NY: Consumers Union, May 2000), <www.consumersunion.org>. National Academy of Sciences, "Major Advances in Biology Should Be Used to Assess Birth Defects From Toxic Chemicals," press release (Washington, DC: 1 June 2000); and Sheila Kaplan and Jim Morris, "Kids at Risk," *U.S. News and World Report*, 19 June 2000.

56. "Agreement Reached on Elimination of Dursban Pesticide for Nearly All Household Uses," *EPA Headlines*, 8 June 2000. U.S. EPA, op. cit. note 53; and Kaplan and Morris, op. cit. note 55.

57. Global use from Pimentel, op. cit. note 44; and from D. Pimentel and D. Kahn, "Environmental Aspects of Cosmetic Standards of Foods and Pesticides," in David Pimentel, ed., *Techniques for Reducing Pesticide Use: Economic and Environmental Benefits* (New York: John Wiley & Sons, 1997). Value from FAO, *FAOSTAT Statistics Database* <apps.fao.org>, viewed 17 December 1999. Toxicity from Polly Short and Theo Colborn, "Pesticide Use in the U.S. and Policy Implications: A Focus on Herbicides," *Toxicology and Industrial Health*, January–March 1999.

58. Pesticides Trust, "The Pesticide Business—Impact on Food Security," <www.gn.apc.org/pesticidestrust/articles/pn42p4.htm>, viewed 6 June 1999; and Short and Colborn, op. cit. note 57. Figure 4 from Sarah Porter, "Pesticide Trade Nears New High," in Brown, Renner, and Haweil, op. cit. note 34.

59. Fatalities from Brian Halweil, "Where Have All the Farmers Gone?" *World Watch*, September/October 2000. Health effects from Robert Repetto and Sanjay S. Baliga, *Pesticides and the Immune System: The Public Health Risks* (Washington, DC: World Resources Institute, March 1996); E. Tielemans et al., "Pesticide Exposure and Decreased Fertilisation Rates in Vitro," *The Lancet*, 7 August 1999; Lennart Hardell and Mikael Eriksson, "A Case-Control Study of Non-Hodgkin Lymphona and Exposure to Pesticides," *Cancer*, 15 March 1999; Vincent F. Garry et al., "Pesticide Appliers, Biocides, and Birth Defects in Rural Minnesota," *Environmental Health Perspectives*, April 1996; Ida S. Weidner et al., "Cryptorchidism and Hypospadias in Sons of Gardeners and Farmers," *Environmental Health Perspectives*, December 1998 (additional information on birth defects); and J. Vena et al., "Exposure to Dioxin and Nonneoplastic Mortality in the Expanded IARC International Cohort Study of Phenoxy Herbicide and Chlorophenol Production Workers and Sprayers," *Environmental Health Perspectives*, April 1998 (heart disease).

60. Bird estimate from Joel Bourne, "Bugging out," *Audubon*, March–April 1999. Alligators from Louis J. Guillette et al., "Developmental Abnormalities of the Gonad and Abnormal Sex Hormone Concentrations in Juvenile Alligators from Contaminated and Control Lakes in Florida," *Environmental Health Perspectives*, August 1994; and Peter M. Vonier et al., "Interaction of Environmental Chemicals with the Estrogen and Progesterone Receptors from the Oviduct of the American Alligator," *Environmental Health Perspectives*, December 1996. Eagles and fish from Weybridge Report, "European Workshop on the Impact of Endocrine Disrupters on Human Health and Wildlife, 2–4 December 1996, Weybridge, U.K.: Report of the Proceedings," (Copenhagen: European Commission DG XII, 16 April 1997); and Marla Cone, "Hormone Study Finds No Firm Answers," *Los Angeles Times*, 4 August 1999. Vultures from Arnab Ray Ghatak, "What's Eating the Vulture?" *Down to Earth*, 15 January 1999. Forests from Thornton, op. cit. note 2.

61. Fred Gould, "The Evolutionary Potential of Crop Pests," *American Scientist*, November–December 1991; Brian Halweil, "Pesticide-Resistant

Species Flourish," in Lester R. Brown, Michael Renner, and Brian Halweil, *Vital Signs 1999* (New York: W.W. Norton & Company, 1999).

62. DDT from Carson, op. cit. note 45. Current levels of resistance and Figure 5 from Halweil, op. cit. note 61.

63. Miguel Altieri, "Escaping the Treadmill," *Ceres*, July/August 1995; FAO, "Organic Agriculture: Item 8 of the Provisional Agenda," Committee on Agriculture, Fifteenth Session, Rome, 25–29 January 1999, <www.fao.org/docrep/meeting/X0075e.htm>, viewed 3 February 2000.

64. Carol Kaesuk Yoon, "Simple Method Found to Increase Crop Yields Vastly," *New York Times*, 22 August 2000; and Youyong Zhu, "Genetic Diversity and Disease Control in Rice," *Nature*, 17 August 2000. Gary Gardner, "IPM and the War on Pests," *World Watch*, March/April 1996. U.S. Midwest from Rick Welsh, *The Economics of Organic Grain and Soybean Production in the Midwestern United States*, Policy Studies Report No. 13 (Greenbelt, MD: Henry A. Wallace Institute of Alternative Agriculture, May 1999).

65. FAO, op. cit. note 63.

66. Chrysanthemum from Amdur, Doull, and Klaassen, op. cit. note 1; and Pimentel, op. cit. note 44. Jan A. Rozendaal, *Vector Control: Methods for Use by Individuals and Communities* (Geneva: WHO, 1997); and Christian Back, "The Use of Persistent Organic Pollutants (POPs) for Vector Control," in *International Experts Meeting on Persistent Organic Pollutants: Towards Global Action*, op. cit. note 47.

67. *Brassica* from J. Raloff, "Coming: A New Crop of Organic Pesticides," *Science News*, 9 October 1999. Insects from Bourne, op. cit. note 60.

68. Stephen Day, "The Sweet Smell of Death," *New Scientist*, 7 September 1996; and Charles M. Benbrook et al., *Pest Management at the Crossroads* (Yonkers, New York: Consumers Union, 1996).

69. Nguyen Huu Dung et al., *Impact of Agro-Chemical Use on Productivity and Health in Vietnam*, Economy and Environment Program for Southeast Asia Research Report Series (Singapore: EEPSEA, January 1999); Barbara Dinham and Dorothy Myers, "Networking for Organic Cotton," *Pesticides News*, December 1997.

70. Helga Willer and Minou Yussefi, "Organic Agriculture World-Wide: Statistics and Perspectives," (Bad Dürkheim: Stiftung, Ökologie & Landbau, 2000). China from Jiang Bin and Er Dong, "Green Future in Store for Organic Food," *China Daily*, 20 December 1999, and from Organic Trade Association (OTA), "Organic Agriculture International Statistics/Info" (Greenfield, MA: OTA, undated), facsimile to Brian Halweil, Worldwatch Institute, received 28 January 2000.

71. $22 billion from Brian Halweil, "Organic Farming Thrives Worldwide," in Brown, Renner, and Halweil, op. cit. note 34. U.S. trade from Barbara Haumann, OTA, Greenfield, MA, e-mail to author, 16 August 2000; U.S. supermarkets from Sandra Gordon, "A Healthy Market," *Kansas City Star*, 14 May 2000; Japan and companies from Willer and Yussefi, op. cit. note 70.

72. Twenty percent margin from FAO, op. cit. note 63. Markets in Nikki van der Gaag, "Pick Your Poison," *New Internationalist*, May 2000. UNCTAD cited in Willer and Yussefi, op. cit. note 70.

73. Rozendaal, op. cit. note 66. WHO, *World Health Organization Report on Infectious Diseases: Removing Obstacles to Healthy Development* (Geneva: 1999); and "Malariasphere," *New Scientist*, 15 July 2000. Unreported deaths from B. Greenwood, "Malaria Mortality and Morbidity in Africa," *Bulletin of the World Health Organization*, vol. 77, no. 8 (1999).

74. "Malariasphere," op. cit. note 73.

75. WWF-U.S., *Resolving the DDT Dilemma: Protecting Human Health and Biodiversity* (Washington, DC: June 1998); and Henk Bouwman, "Malaria Control and the Paradox of DDT," *Africa—Environment and Wildlife*, May 2000.

76. WHO Expert Committee on Malaria, *Twentieth Report*, Technical Report 892 (Geneva: WHO, 2000); WHO, op. cit. note 73.

77. Graham Brown, "Fighting Malaria," *British Medical Journal*, 14 June 1997. Table 3 from WWF, op. cit. note 48.

78. Back, op. cit. note 66.

79. Geoffrey A.T. Target and Brian M. Greenwood, "Impregnated Bednets," *World Health*, May–June 1998. Costs from WHO, op. cit. note 73. F. Chandre, et al., "Status of Pyrethroid Resistance in *Anopheles gambiae* Sensu Lato," *Bulletin of the World Health Organization*, vol. 77, no. 3 (1999).

80. Andy Coghlan, "Four-Pronged Attack," *New Scientist*, 20 February 1999.

81. "Malariasphere," op. cit. note 73.

82. Vinyl Institute web site, <www.vinylinfo.org/materialvinyl/serving-moretour/4monomertopolymer.html>, viewed 13 June 2000; Aida M. Jebens, "Polyvinyl Chloride (PVC) Resins," *CEH (Chemical Economics Handbook) Marketing Research Report* (Zurich: SRI International, 1997); and Principia Partners, "Post-Industrial and Post-Consumer Vinyl Reclaim: Material Flow and Uses in North America," final report to Chlor-Vinyl Steering Group (Exton, PA: July 1999).

83. Year of first production from Thornton, op. cit. note 2; current production from Maack Business Services, "PVC Updates: Supply/Demand," *PVC Insight*, vol. 8, no. 16 (2000); 2 percent from Joel A. Tickner, *Trends in World PVC Industry Expansion*, Greenpeace USA White Paper (Washington, DC: 19 June 1998); 2005 estimate based on rate in "Chemical Market Associates Inc.'s Industry Report," *PVC Insight*, vol. 8, no. 19 (2000). Figure 6 from Jebens, op. cit. note 82 (consumption); and "Polyvinyl Chloride," *PVC Insight*, vol. 8, no. 15 (2000) (production capacity).

84. Half of near-term growth from T. Waltermire, "The Vinyl Plastics Industry," presentation at the Goldman Sachs Fourth Annual Chemical Investor Forum, New York, May 1996. Japan, South Korea, and Taiwan from "Production: Gains Beat Losses: Asia," *Chemical and Engineering News*, 26 June 2000. China's imports from "Chemical Market Associates Inc.'s Industry Report," op. cit. note 83. Asian demand from "Philippine Demand Prompting PVC Capacity Increases," *PVC Insight*, vol. 8, no. 22 (2000); "Tosoh's GM Strategy on PVC Market Scope," ibid.; and "Clinton Releases China Details," *PVC Insight*, vol. 8, no. 18 (2000).

85. "Japan, PVC Output Falls 3.5% in May," *PVC Insight*, vol. 8, no. 21 (2000); "Chemical Market Associates Inc.'s Industry Report," op. cit. note 83; and Jebens, op. cit. note 82.

86. Cumulative estimate from Witze van der Naald and Beverly Thorpe, *PVC Plastic: A Looming Waste Crisis* (Amsterdam: Greenpeace International 1998); in-use estimate based on life-span from Jebens, op. cit. note 82; and Ayres, op. cit. note 27.

87. Pat Costner, scientist, Greenpeace International, e-mail to author, 18 December 1999.

88. Vinyl Institute, op. cit. note 82.

89. EDC process from Environment Agency, *Regulation of Dioxin Releases fom the Runcorn Operations of ICI and EVC* (Warrington, U.K.: January 1997); and Thornton, op. cit. note 2. Production capacity from "Production: Gains Beat Losses," *Chemical and Engineering News*, 26 June 2000; and "Ethylene Dichloride Capacity," *Chemical Week*, 12 March 1997. Health effects from International Safety Chemical Cards, "1-2 Dichloroethane," <www.cdc.gov/niosh/ipcsneng/neng0250.html>, viewed 13 October 2000; and National Safety Council, <www.crossroads.nsc.org/ChemicalTemplate. cfm>, viewed 20 August 2000. Hazard ranking from Environmental Defense, "Chemical Scorecard," available at <www.scorecard.org/chemicalprofiles/summary. tcl?edf_substance_id=107%2d06%2d2>, viewed 22 August 2000.

90. Four kilograms from Thornton, op. cit. note 2. Light and heavy ends from Environment Agency, op. cit. note 89. Identified byproducts from ICI Chemicals and Polymers Ltd., *Report to the Chief Inspector HMIP Authorization AK6039, Improvement Condition, Part 8, Table 8.1, Item 2: Formation of Dioxins in Oxychlorination, Significance for Human Health and Monitoring Proposals*

(Runcorn, U.K.: ICI, Safety and Environment Department, 27 April 1994).

91. Vulcan materials from Pat Costner et al., *PVC: A Principal Contributor to the U.S. Dioxin Burden* (Washington, DC; Greenpeace USA, 1995). PCBs from Dow Chemical, "Heavy Ends from the Distillation of Ethylene Dichloride in Ethylene Dichloride Production," *Waste Analysis Sheet*, revised (Plaquemine, LA: Dow Chemical, March 1991); several tons from Thornton, op. cit. note 2.

92. VCM from ATSDR (Agency for Toxic Substances and Disease Registry) toxicological profile <www.atsdr.cdc.gov/ToxProfiles/phs8825.html>, viewed 12 October 2000; and International Chemical Safety Cards, "Vinyl Chloride," <www.cdc.gov/niosh/ipcsneng/neng0082.html>. Byproduct generation from R. Papp, "Organochlorine Waste Management," *Pure and Applied Chemistry*, vol. 68 no. 9 (1996). VCM production was 22.8 million tons in 1996, the most recent year for which data were available: see Tickner, op. cit. note 83. Russia from F. Khizbullia et al., "Evaluation of Polychlorinated Dibenzofurans Emissions from Vinylchloride-Monomer Production," *Organohalogen Compounds*, vol. 26 (1998), 225-229.

93. Jebens, op. cit. note 82; and Vinyl Institute, op. cit. note 82.

94. Comparison of PVC and other plastics from Stephen Fenichell, *Plastic: The Making of a Synthetic Century* (New York: Harper-Business, 1996); and Joel A. Tickner, Research Associate, Lowell Center for Sustainable Production, University of Massachusetts-Lowell, e-mail to author 26 June 2000. Institute for Local Self-Reliance (ILSR), "Biochemical Plasticizers," *Pollution Solutions*, fact sheet no. 16 (Minneapolis, MN: ILSR, 1996).

95. Amdur, Doull, and Klaassen, op. cit. note 1; and Schettler et al., op. cit. note 3.

96. Robert E. Menzer, "Water and Soil Pollutants," in Amdur, Doull, and Klaassen, op. cit. note 1. Global estimate based on rate derived from Thornton, op. cit. note 2; and data from Catherine A. Harris et al., "The Estrogenic Activity of Phthalates Esters *In Vitro*," *Environmental Health Perspectives*, August 1997; and Schettler et al., op. cit. note 3. Lab materials from <www.ourstolenfuture.org/NewScience/oncompounds/phthalates>, viewed 18 September 2000.

97. Health effects from Schettler et al., op. cit. note 3; European Commission, Director General III, "Ban of Phthalates in Childcare Articles and Toys," press release (Brussels: 10 November 1999), <europa.eu.int/comm/dg03/press/1999/IP99829.htm>, viewed 18 October 2000; and Environmental Data Interactive Exchange, "EC Publishes Details for Emergency Phthalates Ban," 11 December 1999, <www.edie.net/library>, viewed 18 October 2000. Chick embryo and blood bags from Menzer, op. cit. note 96.

98. L.E. Grey et al., "Administration of Potentially Antiandrogenic

Pesticides (Procymidone, Linuron, Iprodione, Chlozolinate, *p,p'*-DDE, and Ketoconazole) and Toxic Substances (Dibutyl- and Diethylhexyl Phthalate, PCB 169, and Ethane Dimethane Sulphonate) During Sexual Differentiation Produces Diverse Profiles of Reproductive Malformations in the Male Rat," *Toxicology and Industrial Health*, vol. 15 (1999), 94–118.

99. No safe level and toy studies from European Commission, op. cit. note 97. Stephen D. Pearson and Lawrence A. Trissel, "Leaching of Diethylhexyl Phthalate from Polyvinyl Chloride Containers by Selected Drugs and Formulation Components," *American Journal of Hospital Pharmacology*, July 1993; Benjamin C. Blount et al., "Levels of Seven Urinary Phthalates Metabolites in a Human Reference Population," *Environmental Health Perspectives*, October 2000.

100. C.G. Ohlson and L. Hardell, "Testicular Cancer and Occupational Exposures with a Focus on Xenoestrogens in Polyvinyl Chloride Plastics," *Chemosphere*, May–June 2000; Ivelisse Colón et al., "Identification of Phthalate Esters in the Serum of Young Puerto Rican Girls with Premature Breast Development," *Environmental Health Perspectives*, September 2000; Jouni J.K. Jaakkola et al., "Interior Surface Materials in the Home and the Development of Bronchial Obstruction in Young Children in Oslo, Norway," *American Journal of Public Health*, February 1999.

101. Eckhard Plincke et al., "Mechanical Recycling of PVC Wastes," Study for DG XI of the European Commission (Basel: Prognos Institute, January 2000) <www.europa.eu.int/comm/environment/waste/report8.pdf>, viewed 15 August 2000.

102. Plincke et al., op. cit. note 101; and Ayres, op. cit. note 27.

103. Products from "Pursuing Better PVCs," *Environmental Health Perspectives*, December 1997; two-thirds from Ayres, op. cit. note 27. Association of Postconsumer Plastic Recyclers, "APPR Takes a Stand on PVC," press release, 15 April 1998.

104. Barbara Stewart, "Workers Pick Up Where New Yorkers' Recycling Leaves Off," *New York Times*, 27 June 2000; 94 percent from Ron Perkins and Barbara Halpin, "Breaking Bottlenecks in Plastic Bottle Recovery," *Resource Recycling*, June 2000; 0.1 percent from Principia Partners, op. cit. note 82; 3 percent from Greenpeace International, "European Commission Studies Confirm PVC Hazards: Greenpeace Calls for Full Phase Out," press release (Brussels: 12 April 2000); export of waste PVC from Greenpeace, "Greenpeace Denounces Toxic PVC-Waste Dumping Plans in Goa," press release (Amsterdam: 4 May 2000); and Health Care Without Harm, "Fact Sheet on Recycling PVC Medical Products," viewed at <www.noharm. org/library/admin/>, 12 October 2000.

105. Argus et al., "The Behaviour of PVC in Landfill," (Brussels: February 2000), available online at <www.europa.eu.int/comm/environment/waste/

report7.pdf>. Japan from Pat Costner, *Dioxin Elimination: A Global Imperative* (Amsterdam: Greenpeace International, 8 March 2000). Chlorine content from Bertin Technologies et al., "The Influence of PVC on the Quantity and Hazardousness of Flue Gas Cleaning Residues from Incineration," (Brussels: April 2000) available at <www.europa.eu.int/comm/environment/waste/report6.pdf>; and Ayres, op. cit. note 27.

106. Argus et al., op. cit. note 105.

107. UNEP Chemicals Division, op. cit. note 5.

108. Mari Yamaguchi, "Japan Facing Dioxin Pollution Woes," *Associated Press*, 3 July 1999; Andrew Pollack, "In Japan's Burnt Trash, Dioxin Threat," *New York Times*, 27 April 1997; other countries from UNEP Chemicals Division, op. cit. note 5; and Heidi Fiedler, UNEP Chemicals Division, Geneva, e-mail to author, 7 October 1999. Quote from Dick Russell, "Health Problem at the Health Care Industry," *The Amicus Journal*, winter 2000.

109. Rebecca Renner, "Backyard Burners Make Up 50% of Dioxin Emissions in Mexico, NAFTA Researchers Find," *Environmental Science & Technology*, 1 March 2000; Kenneth M. Aldous, "Emissions of Polychlorinated Dibenzo-p-dioxins and Polychlorinated Dibenzofurans from the Open Burning of Household Waste in Barrels," *Environmental Science & Technology*, vol. 34, no. 3 (2000); and Rebecca Renner, "Trash Study Creates a Stir, But Little Action," *Environmental Science & Technology*, 1 March 2000; Philippines from Radha Basu, "Landmark Law to Throw Out Waste Incineration," *Inter Press Service*, 7 May 1999; and Von Hernandez, Toxics Campaign Southeast Asia, Greenpeace International, message posted on IPEN e-mail discussion group <pops-network@igc.org>, 18 May 1999.

110. Controversy from Caspar Henderson, "Might PVC Be PC After All?" *Financial Times*, 7 June 2000; EPA, Office of Research and Development, National Center for Environmental Assessment, *Draft Exposure and Human Health Reassessment of 2,3,7,8-Tetrachlorodibenzo-p-Dioxin (TCDD) and Related Compounds*, "Part I: Estimating Exposure to Dioxin-Like Compounds, Volume 2: Sources of Dioxin-Like Compounds in the United States, Chapter 2: Mechanisms of Formation of Dioxin-Like Compounds During Combustion of Organic Materials," (Washington, DC: EPA, March 2000), <www.epa.gov/ncea/pdfs/dioxin/part1and2.htm>, viewed 22 August 2000; and Ayres, op. cit. note 27. Combustion variables from Bertin Technologies et al., op. cit. note 105. German EPA from Thornton, op. cit. note 2.

111. Table 4 from CHEMinfo Services, Inc., "Chapter 10- PVC Products and Markets," in *A Technical & Socio-Economic Comparison of Options, Part 2—Polyvinyl Chloride*, report prepared for Environment Canada (Toronto: November 1997), <www.cciw.ca/glimr/data/chlor-alkali/chap10.html>, viewed 10 May 2000.

112. Soybean oil from ILSR, op. cit. note 94; 15 percent from "Biochemical

Substitutions in the Polymer Industry," ILSR Pollution Solution Fact Sheet no. 4 (Minneapolis: ILSR, 1995).

113. "ReBase Products Offer Solution to Plastics Industry's PVC Problem," *Canadian Chemical News*, November 1999.

114. Greenpeace International, *Chlorine and PVC Restrictions and PVC-Free Policies: A List Compiled by Greenpeace International*, 3rd ed. (Amsterdam: August 1999); Frederick C. Gross and Joe A. Colony, "The Ubiquitous Nature and Objectionable Characteristics of Phthalate Esters in Aerospace Technology," *Environmental Health Perspectives*, January 1973.

115. Joel Tickner, "A Review of the Availability of Plastic Substitutes for Soft PVC in Toys," technical briefing commissioned by Greenpeace International (Lowell, MA: University of Massachusetts, February 1999); cost from Tellus Institute for Resource and Environmental Strategies, CSG/Tellus Packaging Study, *Report #5: Executive Summary*, prepared for the Council of State Governments, U.S. EPA, and the New Jersey Department of Environmental Protection and Energy (Boston: Tellus Institute, May 1992).

116. Jebens, op. cit. note 82; and van der Naald and Thorpe, op. cit. note 86.

117. *Gutta percha* from Meikle, op. cit. note 1. Biopolymers from "Corn Checkoff Pays Off with Plastics Plant," NCGA, 26 April 2000, <www.ncga.com/01hot_off_the_cob/reports/042600.htm>, viewed 7 August 2000; Kim Stelson, University of Minnesota, Department of Mechanical Engineering, conversation with Ann Hwang, Worldwatch Institute, 29 June 2000; Allison Schelesinger, "Perfecting Planet-Friendly Plastics," *IT: Inventing Tomorrow*, (University of Minnesota, Institute of Technology) spring 1999; Tillman U. Gerngross and Steven C. Slater, "How Green Are Green Plastics?" *Scientific American*, August 2000.

118. Stelson, op. cit. note 117; and Gerngross and Slater, op. cit. note 117.

119. Ken Geiser, "Cleaner Production and the Precautionary Principle," in Raffensperger and Tickner, op. cit. note 18; and Joel A. Tickner, "A Map Toward Precautionary Decision Making," in ibid.

120. Töpfer quote from UNEP, "Report," op. cit. note 6; Sara Thurin Rollin, "Fourth Round of POPs Negotiations Closes With Dioxin, Other Major Issues Unresolved," *International Environment Reporter*, 29 March 2000; UNEP, "Preparation of an International Legally Binding Instrument for Implementing International Action on Certain Persistent Organic Pollutants," Draft Text by the Chair, Fifth Session, Johannesburg, 4–9 December 2000, Item 4 of the provisional agenda, (Geneva: 3 August 2000).

121. IPEN scorecard, <www.ipen.org>, viewed 20 September 2000; "Support for Top Issues Tallied," *International Environment Reporter*, 29 March 2000; Lara Santoro, "Banning vs. Managing 'Dirty Dozen' Pollutants," *Christian*

Science Monitor, 16 February 1999; "Leaked Letter Reveals U.S. Threat to Thwart Toxics Treaty," *Environmental News Service*, 3 February 2000.

122. OSPAR, op. cit. note 15.

123. UNEP, "Report of the Intergovernmental Negotiating Committee for an International Legally Binding Instrument for Implementing International Action on Certain Persistent Organic Pollutants on the Work of Its Fourth Session," (Geneva: 25 March 2000), <www.irptc.unep.ch/pops>, viewed 20 September 2000; and WWF, Global Toxic Chemicals Initiative, "UNEP Global POPs Treaty, INC5/Johannesburg: Core Issues Statement," (Washington, DC: WWF, June 2000), <www.ipen.org>, viewed 20 September 2000.

124. Sara Thurin Rollin, "Several Numerical Criteria Set for Adding Chemicals to U.N. Pops Treaty, Officials Say," *International Environment Reporter*, 9 December 1998; IISD, "Report of the First Session of the Criteria Expert Group for Persistent Organic Pollutants: 26–30 October 1998," *Earth Negotiations Bulletin*, 2 November 1998. Table 5 from the following. Aarhus from UNEP, *Analysis of Selected Conventions Covering the Ten Intentionally Produced Persistent Organic Pollutants* (Geneva: 2 June 1999); Daniel Pruzin, "UN/ECE Draft Protocol on Heavy Metals, Persistent Organic Pollutants Concluded," *International Environment Reporter*, 18 February 1998; J. Raloff, "Persistent Pollutants Face Global Ban," *Science News*, 4 July 1998; current status of Aarhus from <www.unece.org/env/lrtap/welcome.html>, viewed 12 October 2000. Rotterdam PIC procedure from FAO, "Rotterdam Convention on Harmful Chemicals and Pesticides Adopted and Signed," press release (Rome: 11 September 1998); UNEP and FAO, "Final Act of the Conference of Plenipotentiaries on the Convention on the Prior Informed Consent Procedure for Certain Hazardous Chemicals and Pesticides in International Trade, Rotterdam, 10–11 September 1998," (Rome: 17 September 1998); current status of PIC from <www.pic.int/finale.htm#convention_text_e>, viewed 20 October 2000. Basel from Basel Action Network (BAN), "The Basel Ban: A Triumph for Global Environmental Justice," Briefing Paper No. 1 (Seattle: BAN, 1 October 1997); FAO, "Rotterdam Convention" op. cit. this note; current status of Basel from Basel Secretariat, UNEP, <www.unep.ch/basel>, viewed 14 October 2000. Table 6 from UNEP, Chemicals Division, *Master List of Actions on the Reduction and/or Elimination of the Releases of Persistent Organic Pollutants*, 2nd ed. (Geneva: February 2000); UNEP, *Summary of Existing National Legislation on persistent Organic Pollutants* (Geneva: 14 June 1999); PCBs specifically from Joint Canada-Philippines Planning Committee, *International Experts Meeting on Persistent Organic Pollutants: Towards Global Action*, meeting background report, Vancouver, Canada, 4–8 June 1995 (revised October 1995); import bans from UNEP and FAO, *Report on Study on International Trade in Widely Prohibited Chemicals* (Rome: 16 February 1996).

125. Eva Webster, Don MacKay, and Frank Wania, "Evaluating Environmental Persistence," *Environmental Toxicology and Chemistry*, vol. 17 no. 11 (1998).

126. Bruce D. Rodan et al., "Screening for Persistent Organic Pollutants: Techniques to Provide a Scientific Basis for POPs Criteria in International Negotiations," *Environmental Science & Technology*, 15 October 1999; chemicals on Aarhus list from UNEP, *Analysis*, op. cit. note 124; and <www.unece.org/env/lrtap/welcome.html>, op. cit. note 124.

127. Lindh cited on Greenpeace Toxics Campaign, "PVC Free Solutions: PVC-Free Initiatives," <www.greenpeace.org/%7Etoxics/toxic_1.html>, viewed 27 September 2000.

128. Basu, op. cit. note 109, and Von Hernandez, op. cit. note 109.

129. Greenpeace International, "European Parliament Demands Full Ban on Soft PVC Toys," press release (Brussels: 7 July 2000); European Commission, op. cit. note 97; Maria Burke, "Phthalate Standard Endorsed by Industry," *Environmental Science & Technology*, 1 October 1999; and Samer Iskander and Emma Tucker, "France Bans 'Toxic' Toys," *Financial Times*, 8 July 1999.

130. More than 100 countries from BAN, op. cit. note 124; PIC from UNEP and FAO, "Final Act," op. cit. note 124; Basel from Basel Secretariat, op. cit. note 124.

131. PIC from UNEP and FAO, "Final Act," op. cit. note 124; Basel from Basel Secretariat, op. cit. note 124; illegal shipments from BAN, op. cit. note 124.

132. Michael Gregory et al., "Issue Topic: Information Exchange and Public Right to Know, Treaty Sections Articles G and H, UNEP Global POPs Treaty (INC5/Johannesburg, December 2000)—POPs and Right to Know," <www.ipen.org>, viewed 20 September 2000; U.S. EPA, "Chapter 1: Toxics Release Inventory Reporting and the 1997 Public Data Release," *Toxics Release Inventory* (Washington, DC: 1997); U.S. EPA, Toxics Release Inventory, <www.epa.gov/tri/general.htm>, viewed 6 August 1999; U.S. General Accounting Office, *Toxic Chemicals: EPA's Toxic Release Inventory Is Useful but Can Be Improved* (Washington, DC: June 1991).

133. Countries from U.S. EPA, Chapter 1, op. cit. note 132; UNEP Chemicals Division, *National Inventories of Persistent Organic Pollutants: Selected Examples as Possible Models*, Preliminary Report (Geneva: July 1999); Jindrich Petrlik, Deti Zeme (Children of the Earth), Prague, message posted on IPEN e-mail discussion group <pops-network@igc.org>, 20 June 1999 (Czech Republic); and UNEP, "National PRTR Activities: Challenges and Experiences," 1 March 1996, <irptc.unep.ch/prtr/nat01.html>, viewed 11 August 1999. "The Citizens Right to Know," *New York Times*, 1 June 1999.

134. Tickner, op. cit. note 119; Beverly Thorpe, *A Citizen's Guide to Clean Production* (Lowell, MA: Center for Clean Products and Clean Technologies, University of Tennessee-Knoxville, and the Lowell Center for Sustainable Production, University of Massachusetts-Lowell, August 1999);

Massachusetts Department of Environmental Protection (DEP), Bureau of Waste Prevention, *1997 Toxics Use Reduction Information Release* (Boston: DEP, 23 March 1999); and Randi Currier and Christopher E. Van Atten, *Benefit-Cost Analysis of the Massachusetts Toxics Use Reduction Act*, Methods and Policy Report 15 (Lowell, MA: Massachusetts Toxics Use Reduction Institute, February 1997).

135. DEP, op. cit. note 134: based on a survey of facilities subject to TURA, economic benefits to the state were $90.5 million between 1990 and 1997, outweighing costs of $76.7 during the same period, exclusive of human health and ecological benefits. See also <www.turi.org/HTMLSrc/turinews. html#TURI>, viewed 21 September 2000. Figure 7 from DEP, op. cit. note 134.

136. Pat Costner, scientist, Greenpeace International, conversation with author, 13 April 2000. For list of participating organizations, see <www.ipen.org>.

137. David S. Hilzenrath, "Nike to Stop Using PVC in Shoes," *Washington Post*, 26 August 1998; Philippines from Basu, op. cit. note 109; Nike, Lego, and IKEA from Greenpeace International, op. cit. note 114; Meagan Boltwood, "PVC: Going, Going, Gone?" *E Magazine*, May/June 1999; Greenpeace International, "General Motors Announces Plan to Go PVC-Free, Breaking Industry Code of Silence on PVC Problems," press release (Amsterdam: 23 September 1999); and "Universal Health Services Leads the Way for Vinyl Phase Out," *Chemical Business Newsbase*, 25 May 1999.

138. David Brown and Caroline E. Mayer, "3M to Pare Scotchgard Products," *Washington Post*, 17 May 2000; "3M and EPA," <www.epa.gov/ opptintr/pbt/whatsnew.htm>, viewed 25 May 2000; and "3M's Big Cleanup: Why It Decided to Pull the Plug on Its Best-Selling Stain Repellant," *BusinessWeek* online, 5 June 2000.

139. "Denmark to Tax PVC and Phthalates," *Greenpeace Business*, August –September 1999.

140. Paper to landfills from Abramovitz and Mattoon, op. cit. note 20.

141. Danish Ministry of Environment and Energy, *Action Plan for Reducing and Phasing Out Phthalates in Soft Plastics* (Copenhagen: June 1999), <www.mst.dk/activi/phthalates%20ngelsk.doc>, viewed 4 October 2000; "Denmark Plans to Cut Phthalates," *Chemical Market Reporter*, 6 July 1999; Anders Emmerman, "Sweden's Reduced Risk Pesticide Policy," *Pesticides News*, December 1996; Olle Pettersson, "Pesticide Use in Swedish Agriculture: The Case of a 75% Reduction," in Pimentel, op. cit. note 57; U.K. Department of the Environment, Transport, and the Regions, "Executive Summary," in *Design of a Tax or Charge Scheme for Pesticides* (London: March 1999); Valerie Frances et al., *F.A.C.T. Fair Agricultural Chemical Taxes: Tax Reform for Sustainable Agriculture* (Washington, DC: Friends of the Earth, May 1999).

142. B. Wahlström and B. Lundqvist, "Risk Reduction and Chemicals Control: Lessons from the Swedish Chemicals Action Programme," in T. Jackson ed., *Clean Production Strategies: Developing Preventive Environmental Management in the Industrial Economy* (Ann Arbor, MI: Lewis, 1993); J.B. Opschoor, "Economic Instruments for Controlling PMPs," in J.B. Opschoor and David Pearce, eds., *Persistent Pollutants: Economics and Policy* (Boston: Kluwer Academic Publishers, 1991); and Thorpe, op. cit. note 134.

Worldwatch Papers

No. of Copies

Worldwatch Papers by Anne Platt McGinn

_____WWP0153 Why Poison Ourselves? A Precautionary Approach to Synthetic Chemicals
_____WWP0145 Safeguarding The Health of Oceans
_____WWP0142 Rocking the Boat: Conserving Fisheries and Protecting Jobs
_____WWP0129 Infecting Ourselves: How Environmental and Social Disruptions Trigger Disease

Climate Change, Energy, and Materials

_____WWP0151 Micropower: The Next Electrical Era
_____WWP0149 Paper Cuts: Recovering the Paper Landscape
_____WWP0144 Mind Over Matter: Recasting the Role of Materials in Our Lives
_____WWP0138 Rising Sun, Gathering Winds: Policies to Stabilize the Climate and
          Strengthen Economies
_____WWP0130 Climate of Hope: New Strategies for Stabilizing the World's Atmosphere
_____WWP0124 A Building Revolution: How Ecology and Health Concerns Are Transforming
          Construction
_____WWP0121 The Next Efficiency Revolution: Creating a Sustainable Materials Economy

Ecological and Human Health

_____WWP0148 Nature's Cornucopia: Our Stake in Plant Diversity
_____WWP0141 Losing Strands in the Web of Life: Vertebrate Declines and the Conservation
          of Biological Diversity
_____WWP0140 Taking a Stand: Cultivating a New Relationship with the World's Forests
_____WWP0128 Imperiled Waters, Impoverished Future: The Decline of Freshwater Ecosystems
_____WWP0120 Net Loss: Fish, Jobs, and the Marine Environment

Economics, Institutions, and Security

_____WWP0152 Working for the Environment: A Growing Source of Jobs
_____WWP0146 Ending Violent Conflict
_____WWP0139 Investing in the Future: Harnessing Private Capital Flows for Environmentally
          Sustainable Development
_____WWP0137 Small Arms, Big Impact: The Next Challenge of Disarmament
_____WWP0134 Getting the Signals Right: Tax Reform to Protect the Environment and the
          Economy
_____WWP0133 Paying the Piper: Subsidies, Politics, and the Environment
_____WWP0127 Eco-Justice: Linking Human Rights and the Environment
_____WWP0126 Partnership for the Planet: An Environmental Agenda for the United Nations
_____WWP0125 The Hour of Departure: Forces That Create Refugees and Migrants
_____WWP0122 Budgeting for Disarmament: The Costs of War and Peace

Food, Water, Population, and Urbanization

_____WWP0150 Underfed and Overfed: The Global Epidemic of Malnutrition
_____WWP0147 Reinventing Cities for People and the Planet
_____WWP0143 Beyond Malthus: Sixteen Dimensions of the Population Problem
_____WWP0136 The Agricultural Link: How Environmental Deterioration Could Disrupt Economic
          Progress
_____WWP0135 Recycling Organic Waste: From Urban Pollutant to Farm Resource
_____WWP0132 Dividing the Waters: Food Security, Ecosystem Health, and the New Politics
          of Scarcity
_____WWP0131 Shrinking Fields: Cropland Loss in a World of Eight Billion

_____Total copies (transfer number to order form on next page)

PUBLICATION ORDER FORM

NOTE: Many Worldwatch publications can be downloaded as PDF files from our website at **www.worldwatch.org**. Orders for printed publications can also be placed on the web.

_____ *State of the World:* **$14.95**
The annual book used by journalists, activists, scholars, and policymakers worldwide to get a clear picture of the environmental problems we face.

_____ **State of the World Library: $30.00 (international subscribers $45)**
Receive *State of the World* and all Worldwatch Papers as they are released during the calendar year.

_____ *Vital Signs:* **$13.00**
The book of trends that are shaping our future in easy-to-read graph and table format, with a brief commentary on each trend.

_____ **WORLD WATCH magazine subscription: $20.00 (international subscribers $35.00)**
Stay abreast of global environmental trends and issues with our award-winning, eminently readable bimonthly magazine.

_____ **Worldwatch Database Disk: $89.00   Check one: ____ PC ____ Mac**
Contains global agricultural, energy, economic, environmental, social, and military indicators from all current Worldwatch publications. Includes *Vital Signs* and *State of the World* as they are published. Disk contains Microsoft Excel spreadsheets 5.0/95 (*.xls) for Windows.

_____ **Worldwatch Papers—See list on previous page Single copy: $5.00**
any combination of titles: 2–5: $4.00 ea. • 6–20: $3.00 ea. • 21 or more: $2.00 ea.

<u>$4.00*</u> Shipping and Handling *($8.00 outside North America)*
minimum charge for S&H; call (800) 555-2028 for bulk order S&H

_____ **TOTAL** (U.S. dollars only)

Make check payable to: Worldwatch Institute, 1776 Massachusetts Ave., NW, Washington, DC 20036-1904 USA

❏ Enclosed is my check or purchase order for U.S. $_____

❏ AMEX ❏ VISA ❏ MasterCard _____
Card Number   Expiration Date

signature _____

name _____ **daytime phone #**

address _____

city   **state**   **zip/country**

phone: (800) 555-2028   fax: (202) 296-7365   e-mail: wwpub@worldwatch.org
website: www.worldwatch.org

Wish to make a tax-deductible contribution? Contact Worldwatch to find out how your donation can help advance our work.

Worldwatch Papers

No. of Copies

Worldwatch Papers by Anne Platt McGinn

_____WWP0153 Why Poison Ourselves? A Precautionary Approach to Synthetic Chemicals
_____WWP0145 Safeguarding The Health of Oceans
_____WWP0142 Rocking the Boat: Conserving Fisheries and Protecting Jobs
_____WWP0129 Infecting Ourselves: How Environmental and Social Disruptions Trigger Disease

Climate Change, Energy, and Materials

_____WWP0151 Micropower: The Next Electrical Era
_____WWP0149 Paper Cuts: Recovering the Paper Landscape
_____WWP0144 Mind Over Matter: Recasting the Role of Materials in Our Lives
_____WWP0138 Rising Sun, Gathering Winds: Policies to Stabilize the Climate and Strengthen Economies
_____WWP0130 Climate of Hope: New Strategies for Stabilizing the World's Atmosphere
_____WWP0124 A Building Revolution: How Ecology and Health Concerns Are Transforming Construction
_____WWP0121 The Next Efficiency Revolution: Creating a Sustainable Materials Economy

Ecological and Human Health

_____WWP0148 Nature's Cornucopia: Our Stake in Plant Diversity
_____WWP0141 Losing Strands in the Web of Life: Vertebrate Declines and the Conservation of Biological Diversity
_____WWP0140 Taking a Stand: Cultivating a New Relationship with the World's Forests
_____WWP0128 Imperiled Waters, Impoverished Future: The Decline of Freshwater Ecosystems
_____WWP0120 Net Loss: Fish, Jobs, and the Marine Environment

Economics, Institutions, and Security

_____WWP0152 Working for the Environment: A Growing Source of Jobs
_____WWP0146 Ending Violent Conflict
_____WWP0139 Investing in the Future: Harnessing Private Capital Flows for Environmentally Sustainable Development
_____WWP0137 Small Arms, Big Impact: The Next Challenge of Disarmament
_____WWP0134 Getting the Signals Right: Tax Reform to Protect the Environment and the Economy
_____WWP0133 Paying the Piper: Subsidies, Politics, and the Environment
_____WWP0127 Eco-Justice: Linking Human Rights and the Environment
_____WWP0126 Partnership for the Planet: An Environmental Agenda for the United Nations
_____WWP0125 The Hour of Departure: Forces That Create Refugees and Migrants
_____WWP0122 Budgeting for Disarmament: The Costs of War and Peace

Food, Water, Population, and Urbanization

_____WWP0150 Underfed and Overfed: The Global Epidemic of Malnutrition
_____WWP0147 Reinventing Cities for People and the Planet
_____WWP0143 Beyond Malthus: Sixteen Dimensions of the Population Problem
_____WWP0136 The Agricultural Link: How Environmental Deterioration Could Disrupt Economic Progress
_____WWP0135 Recycling Organic Waste: From Urban Pollutant to Farm Resource
_____WWP0132 Dividing the Waters: Food Security, Ecosystem Health, and the New Politics of Scarcity
_____WWP0131 Shrinking Fields: Cropland Loss in a World of Eight Billion

_____Total copies (transfer number to order form on next page)

PUBLICATION ORDER FORM

NOTE: Many Worldwatch publications can be downloaded as PDF files from our website at **www.worldwatch.org**. Orders for printed publications can also be placed on the web.

_____ *State of the World:* **$14.95**
The annual book used by journalists, activists, scholars, and policymakers worldwide to get a clear picture of the environmental problems we face.

_____ **State of the World Library: $30.00 (international subscribers $45)**
Receive *State of the World* and all Worldwatch Papers as they are released during the calendar year.

_____ *Vital Signs:* **$13.00**
The book of trends that are shaping our future in easy-to-read graph and table format, with a brief commentary on each trend.

_____ **WORLD WATCH magazine subscription: $20.00 (international subscribers $35.00)**
Stay abreast of global environmental trends and issues with our award-winning, eminently readable bimonthly magazine.

_____ **Worldwatch Database Disk: $89.00   Check one: _____ PC _____ Mac**
Contains global agricultural, energy, economic, environmental, social, and military indicators from all current Worldwatch publications. Includes *Vital Signs* and *State of the World* as they are published. Disk contains Microsoft Excel spreadsheets 5.0/95 (*.xls) for Windows.

_____ **Worldwatch Papers—See list on previous page Single copy: $5.00**
any combination of titles: 2–5: $4.00 ea. • 6–20: $3.00 ea. • 21 or more: $2.00 ea.

$4.00* Shipping and Handling *($8.00 outside North America)*
minimum charge for S&H; call (800) 555-2028 for bulk order S&H

_____ **TOTAL** (U.S. dollars only)

Make check payable to: Worldwatch Institute, 1776 Massachusetts Ave., NW, Washington, DC 20036-1904 USA

❑ Enclosed is my check or purchase order for U.S. $_____

❑ AMEX ❑ VISA ❑ MasterCard _____
                                    Card Number   Expiration Date

signature _____

name _____ **daytime phone #** _____

address _____

city _____ **state** _____ **zip/country** _____

phone: (800) 555-2028   fax: (202) 296-7365   e-mail: wwpub@worldwatch.org
website: www.worldwatch.org

Wish to make a tax-deductible contribution? Contact Worldwatch to find out how your donation can help advance our work.